Orthopedic Nursing:
Caring for Patients with Musculoskeletal Disorders

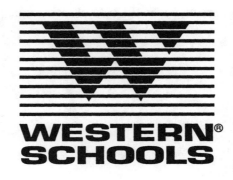

WESTERN® SCHOOLS

By
Dr. Judith A. Halstead

P.O. Box 1930
Brockton, MA 02303
WESTERN SCHOOLS 1-800-438-8888

ABOUT THE AUTHOR

Dr. Judith A. Halstead is Professor of Nursing and Director, Undergraduate Nursing, at USI School of Nursing and Health Professions, in Evansville, Indiana. She has 27 years of experience as a registered nurse, specializing in adult medical-surgical nursing in acute care settings. Dr. Halstead has 24 years of experience as a nurse educator in diploma, associate, baccalaureate, and master's degree nursing programs. She has several years experience in teaching orthopedic nursing to undergraduate nursing students. She is the author of numerous publications, including study guides for medical-surgical nursing, NCLEX review test questions, and case studies in medical-surgical nursing.

Judith Halstead has disclosed that she has no significant financial or other conflicts of interest pertaining to this course book.

ABOUT THE SUBJECT MATTER REVIEWER

Sandra A. Robinson, RN, MSN, CNA, has over eight years experience in the nursing care of orthopedic patients. For the past four years she has served as an educator on faculty at Mississippi College School of Nursing in Clinton, Mississippi. In her role as instructor, she teaches the content related to musculoskeletal disorders and injuries. Her current clinical practice is in the care of orthopedic patients in an acute care setting.

Nurse Planner: Amy Bernard, RN, BSN, MS

Copy Editor: Demi Rasmussen

Indexer: Sylvia Coates

Western Schools' courses are designed to provide nursing professionals with the educational information they need to enhance their career development. The information provided within these course materials is the result of research and consultation with prominent nursing and medical authorities and is, to the best of our knowledge, current and accurate. However, the courses and course materials are provided with the understanding that Western Schools is not engaged in offering legal, nursing, medical, or other professional advice.

Western Schools' courses and course materials are not meant to act as a substitute for seeking out professional advice or conducting individual research. When the information provided in the courses and course materials is applied to individual circumstances, all recommendations must be considered in light of the uniqueness pertaining to each situation.

Western Schools' course materials are intended solely for your use and not for the benefit of providing advice or recommendations to third parties. Western Schools devoids itself of any responsibility for adverse consequences resulting from the failure to seek nursing, medical, or other professional advice. Western Schools further devoids itself of any responsibility for updating or revising any programs or publications presented, published, distributed, or sponsored by Western Schools unless otherwise agreed to as part of an individual purchase contract.

Products (including brand names) mentioned or pictured in Western School's courses are not endorsed by Western Schools, the American Nurses Credentialing Center (ANCC), or any state board.

ISBN: 1-57801-108-6

IMPORTANT: Read these instructions *BEFORE* proceeding!

Enclosed with your course book, you will find the FasTrax® answer sheet. Use this form to answer all the final exam questions that appear in this course book. If you are completing more than one course, be sure to write your answers on the appropriate answer sheet. Full instructions and complete grading details are printed on the FasTrax instruction sheet, also enclosed with your order. Please review them before starting. *If you are mailing your answer sheet(s) to Western Schools, we recommend you make a copy as a backup.*

ABOUT THIS COURSE

A Pretest is provided with each course to test your current knowledge base regarding the subject matter contained within this course. Your Final Exam is a multiple choice examination. **You will find the exam questions at the end of each chapter.**

Use a <u>black</u> pen to fill in your answer sheet.

A PASSING SCORE

You must score 70% or better in order to pass this course and receive your Certificate of Completion. Should you fail to achieve the required score, we will send you an additional FasTrax answer sheet so that you may make a second attempt to pass the course. Western Schools will allow you three chances to pass the same course...*at no extra charge!* After three failed attempts to pass the same course, your file will be closed.

RECORDING YOUR HOURS

Please monitor the time it takes to complete this course using the handy log sheet on the other side of this page. See below for transferring study hours to the course evaluation.

COURSE EVALUATIONS

In this course book, you will find a short evaluation about the course you are soon to complete. This information is vital to providing Western Schools with feedback on this course. The course evaluation answer section is in the lower right hand corner of the FasTrax answer sheet marked "Evaluation," with answers marked 1–22. Your answers are important to us; please take a few minutes to complete the evaluation.

On the back of the FasTrax instruction sheet, there is additional space to make any comments about the course, the school, and suggested new curriculum. Please mail the FasTrax instruction sheet, with your comments, back to Western Schools in the envelope provided with your course order.

TRANSFERRING STUDY TIME

Upon completion of the course, transfer the total study time from your log sheet to question 22 in the course evaluation. The answers will be in ranges; please choose the proper hour range that best represents your study time. You **MUST** log your study time under question 22 on the course evaluation.

EXTENSIONS

You have two (2) years from the date of enrollment to complete this course. A six (6) month extension may be purchased. If after 30 months from the original enrollment date you do not complete the course, *your file will be closed and no certificate can be issued.*

CHANGE OF ADDRESS?

In the event you have moved during the completion of this course, please call our student services department at 1-800-618-1670, and we will update your file.

A GUARANTEE TO WHICH YOU'LL GIVE HIGH HONORS

If any continuing education course fails to meet your expectations or if you are not satisfied in any manner, for any reason, you may return it for an exchange or a refund (less shipping and handling) within 30 days. Software, video, and audio courses must be returned unopened.

Thank you for enrolling at Western Schools!

WESTERN SCHOOLS
P.O. Box 1930
Brockton, MA 02303
(800) 438-8888
www.westernschools.com

Orthopedic Nursing
Caring for Patients
with Musculoskeletal Disorders

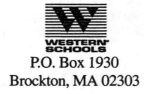

WESTERN
SCHOOLS
P.O. Box 1930
Brockton, MA 02303

Please use this log to total the number of hours you spend reading the text and taking the final examination (use 50-min hours).

Date	Hours Spent
2/10/05	
TOTAL	

Please log your study hours with submission of your final exam. To log your study time, fill in the appropriate circle under question 22 of the FasTrax® answer sheet under the "Evaluation" section.

Orthopedic Nursing
Caring for Patients with Musculoskeletal Disorders

WESTERN SCHOOLS
CONTINUING EDUCATION EVALUATION

Instructions: Mark your answers to the following questions with a black pen on the "Evaluation" section of your FasTrax® answer sheet provided with this course. You should not return this sheet.

Please use the scale below to rate how well the course content met the educational objectives.

A	Agree Strongly	C	Disagree Somewhat
B	Agree Somewhat	D	Disagree Strongly

After completing this course I am able to:

1. Describe the issues relevant to the current practice of orthopedic nursing.

2. Describe the basic anatomy and physiology of the musculoskeletal system.

3. Describe how to perform an assessment of the musculoskeletal system.

4. Describe the clinical manifestations of musculoskeletal disorders.

5. Describe the diagnostic tests used to diagnose disorders of the musculoskeletal system, as well as the nursing care associated with the procedures.

6. Describe the various treatment interventions that are used when caring for patients who have experienced musculoskeletal trauma.

7. Describe the nursing care of patients who have experienced a fracture.

8. Describe the medical management and nursing care of patients who have experienced a fracture of the upper extremity or lower extremity. Also address fractures of the clavicle, pelvis, and spine.

9. Describe the medical management and nursing care of patients who have experienced a fracture of the hip.

10. Describe the medical management and nursing care of patients who have osteomyelitis and, in addition, the prevention of osteomyelitis.

11. Describe the medical management and nursing care of patients who have experienced a musculoskeletal injury.

12. Describe the nursing care of patients who have arthritis. Also discuss rheumatoid arthritis, osteoarthritis (degenerative joint disease), and gout.

13. Describe the nursing care of patients who have osteoporosis. Discuss health promotion activities that can help prevent the development of osteoporosis.

14. Describe the medical management and nursing care of patients who have experienced a total joint replacement.

15. Describe the medical management and nursing care of patients who have a bone neoplasm or tumor and, in addition, the care of a patient who has an amputation.

16. The content of this course was relevant to the objectives.

17. This offering met my professional education needs.

18. The objectives met the overall purpose/goal of the course.

19. The course was generally well-written and the subject matter explained thoroughly. (If no, please explain on the back of the FasTrax instruction sheet.)

20. The content of this course was appropriate for home study.

21. The final examination was well-written and at an appropriate level for the content of the course.

22. **PLEASE LOG YOUR STUDY HOURS WITH SUBMISSION OF YOUR FINAL EXAM.**
    Please choose which best represents the total study hours it took to complete this 30-hour course.

    A. less than 25 hours   C. 29–32 hours
    B. 25–28 hours   D. greater than 32 hours

CONTENTS

FIGURES AND TABLES

PRETEST

1. Begin this course by taking the pretest. Circle the answers to the questions on this page, or write the answers on a separate sheet of paper. Do not log answers to the pretest questions on the FasTrax test sheet included with the course.

2. Compare your answers to the PRETEST KEY located in the back of the book. The pretest answer key indicates the course chapter where the content of that question is discussed. Make note of the questions you missed, so that you can focus on those areas as you complete the course.

3. Complete the course by reading each chapter and completing the exam questions at the end of the chapter. Answers to these exam questions should be logged on the FasTrax test sheet included with the course.

1. An example of a long bone is the
   a. vertebra.
   b. femur.
   c. scapula.
   d. metatarsal.

2. At the neuromuscular junction, muscle fiber receptors are stimulated by
   a. adenosine triphosphate (ATP).
   b. creatine phosphate.
   c. acetylcholine.
   d. calcium ions.

3. A nurse making an assessment may find that the neurological status of an extremity has been impaired if there is
   a. decreased capillary refill time.
   b. erythema.
   c. paresthesia.
   d. edema.

4. The development of osteoporosis can result from long-term use of
   a. aspirin.
   b. corticosteroids.
   c. calcium channel blockers.
   d. diuretics.

5. A patient who has suffered an open fracture is at risk for
   a. muscle atrophy.
   b. osteoarthritis.
   c. contractures.
   d. infection.

6. A priority nursing goal during the acute phase of a fracture injury is
   a. administering antibiotics.
   b. promoting adequate nutrition.
   c. encouraging mobility.
   d. providing pain control.

7. The most common indication of compartment syndrome is

   a. progressive, severe pain unrelieved by analgesics.

   b. edema in the affected extremity.

   c. a sensation of tingling in the affected body part.

   d. loss of function.

8. One of the most common potential complications of a humeral shaft fracture is

   a. the development of a "frozen" shoulder.

   b. compartment syndrome.

   c. radial nerve damage.

   d. shortened arm length.

9. In caring for a newly admitted patient who has a fractured pelvis, the nurse knows to carefully assess the patient for

   a. hypovolemic shock.

   b. hypokalemia.

   c. pulmonary infection.

   d. thrombophlebitis.

10. The diagnostic test most effective for diagnosing of osteomyelitis in its early stages is

    a. arthrocentesis.

    b. standard X-ray.

    c. elevated sedimentation rate.

    d. bone scan.

11. A common complication of osteoporosis is

    a. thrombophlebitis.

    b. bone fracture.

    c. osteoarthritis.

    d. bone cancer.

12. The most common symptom associated with musculoskeletal problems is

    a. loss of function.

    b. joint swelling.

    c. pain.

    d. altered mobility.

13. A patient with a plaster of Paris cast should be instructed to

    a. not get the cast wet.

    b. trim the edges of the cast daily.

    c. use cotton swabs to scratch under the cast.

    d. keep the extremity in a dependent position to decrease pressure points.

14. A condition that can slow the healing process of a fracture is

    a. use of nonsteroidal anti-inflammatory drugs to control pain.

    b. inadequate nutritional intake.

    c. immobilization of the affected body part.

    d. decreased fluid intake.

15. A clinical problem that can lead to the development of compartment syndrome is

    a. improper alignment of a fracture.

    b. onset of an infection in the bone.

    c. circulatory compromise.

    d. muscle atrophy.

16. In providing discharge instructions to a patient who has fractured his clavicle, the nurse should tell the patient

    a. to exercise fingers, wrist and elbow.

    b. not to lie supine until the clavicle has healed.

    c. to perform shoulder "shrugs" every four hours.

    d. to gently lift affected arm over the head daily.

17. One characteristic of an intracapsular hip fracture is that

   a. intracapsular fractures are more common in younger individuals.

   b. avascular necrosis is a potential complication.

   c. intracapsular hip fractures affect the lesser trochanter.

   d. the fracture usually heals rapidly.

18. The most common complication following surgery for a fractured hip is

   a. urinary tract infection.

   b. deep vein thrombosis.

   c. perineal nerve damage.

   d. compartment syndrome.

19. The drug of choice for treating osteoarthritis is

   a. nonsteroidal anti-inflammatories.

   b. aspirin.

   c. acetaminophen.

   d. corticosteroids.

20. After total hip replacement surgery, patients should avoid

   a. lying flat in bed.

   b. elevating the head of the bed 45 degrees.

   c. sitting in a firm chair.

   d. crossing the legs.

21. To be eligible to take the certification examination offered by the Orthopaedic Nurses Certification Board (ONCB), a nurse must

   a. have a Master's degree in nursing.

   b. hold an unrestricted license as a registered nurse.

   c. have three years full-time experience in orthopedic nursing care.

   d. have accrued 30 continuing education units in orthopedic nursing.

22. For a patient who has a fractured femur that is healing, the nurse would expect to find laboratory results indicating

   a. decreased serum calcium.

   b. increased alkaline phosphatase level.

   c. increased serum phosphorus level.

   d. decreased creatine kinase.

23. A strain is most accurately defined as a

   a. tear in skeletal muscle.

   b. bruised bone.

   c. overextended ligament.

   d. torn tendon.

24. For a patient who has recently had an above-the-knee amputation and reports that he can still feel his foot tingling, the nurse should respond

   a. "That is not possible. Your pain medication must be causing you to have hallucinations."

   b. "It will take you awhile to accept the fact that your right leg has been amputated."

   c. "That is called phantom limb sensation. It is normal and will eventually disappear."

   d. "If you will keep your residual limb elevated the feeling will subside."

INTRODUCTION

The purpose of this course is to provide licensed practical nurses and registered nurses with a comprehensive review of the concepts related to the practice of orthopedic nursing and care of patients with musculoskeletal disorders. The content includes a brief overview of the anatomy and physiology of the musculoskeletal system, including age-specific considerations. Nursing assessment skills, diagnostic studies, and therapeutic interventions related to the care of patients who have musculoskeletal disorders are addressed. The course focuses on the nursing management of patients who have common musculoskeletal disorders, including those resulting from trauma, infection, inflammation, degeneration, metabolic bone disease, and neoplasms. The principles of rehabilitation as they related to specific musculoskeletal disorders are also addressed. The goal of this course is to provide nurses interested in orthopedic nursing with increased knowledge about the basic principles of orthopedic nursing practice. This is a 30-hour course.

CHAPTER 1

INTRODUCTION TO ORTHOPEDIC NURSING

CHAPTER OBJECTIVE

After completing this chapter, the reader will be able to describe the issues relevant to the current practice of orthopedic nursing.

LEARNING OBJECTIVES

After studying this chapter, the reader will be able to

1. indicate the historical beginnings of orthopedics and orthopedic nursing.

2. identify societal factors that influence the practice of orthopedic nursing.

3. specify the standards of practice that influence orthopedic nursing care.

4. select professional resources available to orthopedic nurses.

OVERVIEW

The specialty of orthopedic nursing practice focuses on the nursing care of patients who have a musculoskeletal disease or disorder. This chapter provides a brief overview of the beginning of orthopedics as a specialty practice in medicine and nursing, identifying societal factors that are influencing the practice of orthopedic nursing today. The standards of practice related to the practice of orthopedic nursing are discussed. The professional resources available to orthopedic nurses to promote continued professional development are also addressed.

HISTORICAL BEGINNINGS

The term orthopedics comes from two Greek words, "orthos" and "paidos" — "orthos" meaning "straight" and "paidos" meaning "child" — thus "straight child." The origin of this term dates from 1741, when it was coined by Nicholas Andre, who wrote a medical book entitled "Orthopaedia, or The Art of Correcting and Preventing Deformities in Children" (Schoen, 2000). Today, the term refers to the treatment of musculoskeletal problems in patients of any age and has been a recognized specialty in medicine in the United States since the late 19th century.

The first orthopedic institution was established in 1780 in Switzerland. It was almost 100 years later before the specialty practice of orthopedics became established in the United States. One of the first well-known practitioners of orthopedic medicine was Hugh Owen Thomas (1834–1891) from Liverpool, England. Thomas was known for his ability to reduce fractures and dislocated joints. His name is still known in today's practice of orthopedics, as evidenced by the Thomas splint, which is used to provide support to fractures. A pioneer in orthopedic surgery in the United States was Dr. Virgil Gibney, who practiced in New York City as the Surgeon-in-Chief of the New York Hospital for the Ruptured and Crippled. The American Orthopaedic Association, the professional organization for orthopedic surgeons, was established in 1887 (Schoen, 2000).

Orthopedic nursing probably got its start in England. Agnes Hunt (1862–1948) is considered one of the early pioneers in orthopedic nursing and has been referred to as the "Florence Nightingale of orthopedic nursing" (Schoen, 2000). She established a home in Oswestry, England, for patients with orthopedic problems in 1900. Baschurch Home prospered and became a large orthopedic hospital that served as a training ground for many orthopedic nurses.

In the United States, the nursing profession was slow to establish a professional organization for the practice of orthopedic nursing. The first organization, Orthopedic Nurses Association, was started in 1972 but is no longer in existence. The current professional nursing organization is the National Association of Orthopaedic Nurses (NAON), which was established in 1980. The goal of NAON is to promote the professional practice of orthopedic nursing and encourage continuing education (Schoen, 2000). The professional journal associated with orthopedic nursing practice is *Orthopedic Nursing*.

SOCIETAL FACTORS AFFECTING ORTHOPEDIC NURSING PRACTICE

The single biggest factor impacting the practice of orthopedic nursing is likely to be the aging of society. Orthopedic nurses can be found practicing in varied health care settings and caring for patients across the life span. However, the majority of patients seeking health care for musculoskeletal problems are middle-aged or elderly. It is no secret that the population of the United States is aging in record numbers. The incidence of osteoporosis, arthritis, hip fractures, and total joint replacements

is expected to increase in the next decade and beyond as the baby boomers enter their senior years. This increased number of elderly individuals will definitely impact the health care resources of our country and will increase the number of patients seeking medical care and nursing care for musculoskeletal-related health problems.

Another societal factor that affects orthopedic nursing practice are lifestyle choices that impact the health of an individual's musculoskeletal system. There is a significant interest in pursuing physical fitness and sports activities. Running, aerobics, yoga, skiing, and biking are just some of the examples of physical fitness activities that can result in musculoskeletal injury. The increased interest in participation in organized sports such as football, basketball, and soccer also account for increased numbers of younger adults seeking health care for traumatic musculoskeletal injuries suffered while pursuing these sports. On the other hand, the United States also has a large population of sedentary individuals who can be called "weekend warriors," limiting their pursuit of physical fitness to the weekend after a week of sedentary work activity. These individuals are at a particularly high risk of musculoskeletal injury as they tend to overextend the capabilities of their bodies when they do pursue a physical activity. Obesity adds stress to joints and the lack of calcium intake in the diet predisposes many individuals to the development of osteoporosis.

Another factor affecting the practice of orthopedic nursing is the early discharge of patients from acute care settings. As health care systems discharge patients earlier than ever, many patients who are recovering from orthopedic injuries or surgery find themselves discharged to extended care facilities or to their home to continue their recovery. To accommodate the health care needs of these patients, the practice of orthopedic nursing is expanding into long-term care facilities, the community, and ambulatory care clinics.

Advances in technology are also impacting the practice of orthopedics. Surgical techniques, prosthetic device materials, and improved diagnostic imaging have greatly improved the success rate of many orthopedic procedures. Complications that continue to affect patient recovery from orthopedic injuries or surgeries are, for the most part, related to the hazards of immobility or infection. The orthopedic nurse has a primary responsibility to provide or direct the nursing care that prevents the development of these complications.

STANDARDS OF PRACTICE FOR ORTHOPEDIC NURSING

The specialty practice of orthopedic nursing is a challenging one. Orthopedic nursing is defined as the care of individuals who have known or predicted neuromusculoskeletal alterations (Schoen, 2000). To provide quality nursing care, the nurse must consider the patient from a holistic perspective, attending to the physical, psychosocial, and spiritual needs of patients and their families. The nurse in orthopedic practice must be knowledgeable about acute care nursing concepts as well as rehabilitation principles. The orthopedic nurse must also be current in his or her practice of medical-surgical nursing, as many patients with musculoskeletal problems have co-existing health problems that can impact their recovery.

Orthopedic nursing practice, as all nursing care practice, is guided by the Standards of Practice established by the American Nurses Association (ANA). In addition, though, there are Standards of Orthopedic Nursing Practice that have been established by NAON. These standards were first established in 1976 and are revised and updated at periodic intervals. The standards of practice are based on the nursing process.

Nurses specializing in orthopedic nursing have multiple opportunities to practice their specialty.

Many practice in acute care settings. As patients are discharged from the hospital earlier than ever before, however, increasing numbers of orthopedic nurses are employed in rehabilitation facilities, community settings, and home health agencies. Geri Tierney, president-elect of NAON in 2002, stated that orthopedic nurses focus on providing patient education and support to those individuals who are potentially facing significant lifestyle changes. Tierney further stated that the two nursing diagnoses that orthopedic nurses work with most often are those associated with the clinical manifestations of impaired mobility and pain (Spotlight on orthopedic nursing, 2002).

The vast majority of nurses practicing orthopedic nursing have a general background in medical-surgical nursing and develop their expertise in orthopedics with on-the-job training (Nursing 2002). Certification opportunities do exist for registered nurses who practice in orthopedics. To be eligible to take the certification examination that is offered by the Orthopaedic Nurses Certification Board (ONCB), the nurse must hold an unrestricted RN license, have two years experience as a RN, and 1000 hours of orthopedic nursing practice. The national professional specialty organization, NAON, is a source of much information for those who practice orthopedic nursing. The website resource for NAON is http://www.orthonurse.org. See Table 1–1 for additional resources that orthopedic nurses may find helpful to their practice.

OVERVIEW OF COURSE

This course will provide a review of the concepts related to orthopedic nursing practice and the care of patients with common musculoskeletal disorders. The course begins with a brief review of the anatomy and physiology of the musculoskeletal system. The next four chapters address the general concepts of patient care that are related to orthopedic nursing. Assessment of the musculoskeletal system and the most common clinical manifestations of musculoskeletal disorders are addressed, along with diagnostic tests and therapeutic nursing interventions related to the care of patients with musculoskeletal disorders.

The course will focus on the nursing management of patients with musculoskeletal disorders resulting from trauma, infection, inflammation, degeneration, metabolic bone disease, and neoplasms. As many musculoskeletal disorders are chronic in nature or require extended periods of recovery time, the principles of rehabilitation as they relate to specific disorders are addressed. The goal of this course is to provide the nurse who has an interest in orthopedic nursing with increased knowledge about the principles of orthopedic nursing practice.

SUMMARY

This introductory chapter provided an overview on the history of the orthopedics specialty and the societal factors currently affecting orthopedic nursing practice. The Standards of Practice for Orthopedic Nursing were also addressed, as were professional resources available to promote the professional growth of orthopedic nurses.

TABLE 1–1: RESOURCES FOR ORTHOPEDIC NURSES

Professional Organizations

Academy of Medical-Surgical Nurses
  www.medsurgnurse.org/

American Nurses Association
  www.nursingworld.org/

American Association of Orthopaedic Surgeons
  www.aaos.org/

Association of Rehabilitation Nurses
  www.rehabnurse.org/

Canadian Orthopaedic Nurses Association
  www.cona-nurse.org/

National Association of Orthopaedic Nurses
  www.orthonurse.org/

National Association of Orthopaedic Technologists
  www.naot.org/

The Internet Society of Orthopedic Surgery and Trauma
  www. orthogate.com/

Professional Journals

International Journal of Trauma Nursing

Journal of the American Academy of Orthopaedic Surgeons
  www.jaaos.org/

MedSurg Nursing
  www.medsurgnurse.org/

Orthopedic Knowledge Online
  www5.aaos.org/oko/

Orthopedic Nursing Journal
  www.orthonurse.org/

The Journal of Bone and Joint Surgery
  www.ejbjs.org/

Resources for Specific Musculoskeletal Disorders

Arthritis Foundation
  www.arthritis.org/

Bone and Joint Decade 2000-2010
  www.boneandjointdecade.org/

National Institute on Aging
  www.nia.nih.gov/

National Institute of Arthritis and Musculoskeletal and Skin Diseases
  www.niams.nih.gov/

National Institutes of Health, Osteoporosis and Related Bone Diseases — National Resource Center
  www.osteo.org/

National Osteoporosis Foundation
  www.nof.org/

EXAM QUESTIONS

CHAPTER 1
Questions 1–4

1. The first organization in the United States devoted to the specialty of orthopedic nursing was established in

    a. 1890.

    b. 1900.

    c. 1972.

    d. 1980.

2. The societal factor that will likely have the most impact on the practice of orthopedic nursing is the

    a. nursing shortage.

    b. lifestyle choices of individuals.

    c. advances in biotechnology.

    d. aging of the populace.

3. The standards of practice for orthopedic nursing are based on the

    a. nursing process.

    b. ANA's Code of Ethics.

    c. orthopedic certification examination.

    d. Nurse Practice Act.

4. The current national professional organization for orthopedic nursing is the

    a. American Nurses' Association.

    b. National Association of Orthopaedic Nurses.

    c. Orthopedic Nurses Association.

    d. National League for Nursing.

CHAPTER 2

OVERVIEW OF THE MUSCULOSKELETAL SYSTEM: ANATOMY AND PHYSIOLOGY

CHAPTER OBJECTIVE

After completing this chapter, the reader will be able to describe the basic anatomy and physiology of the musculoskeletal system.

LEARNING OBJECTIVES

After studying this chapter, the reader will be able to

1. identify the types, structure and function of bone.

2. differentiate the basic physiologic processes associated with the growth and repair of bone.

3. identify the structure and function of joints, cartilage, ligaments, and tendons.

4. identify the structure and function of skeletal muscle.

5. specify the changes that occur in the musculoskeletal system as a result of the aging process.

OVERVIEW

The musculoskeletal system provides the structure and support through which our body is capable of performing coordinated movements. In addition to providing support and producing movement, the musculoskeletal system also provides a protective covering for vital organs, stores minerals, and plays a role in the production of blood cells. To understand the diseases and disorders of the musculoskeletal system and the nursing care associated with these health problems, the nurse must first have knowledge of normal anatomy and physiology. This chapter provides a review of the anatomy and physiology of bones, joints, cartilage, ligaments, tendons, and muscles. The physiological processes associated with the growth and repair of bones are also addressed. The chapter also addresses changes in the musculoskeletal system that develop as aging occurs.

BONE

Function of Bone

The bones in our body have several functions. They provide structural support and form protective coverings over vital organs. Bones also provide attachment points for muscles, serving as levers to produce movement when the muscles contract. In addition, bones provide a storage area for calcium and phosphorus, and they play a role in the production of blood cells. Bone is a living, dynamic tissue, continually engaged in a growth and reabsorption process (Casteel, 2003; Ruda, 2000a). There are 206 bones in the human skeleton (see Figure 2-1).

Types of Bone

Bone can be classified in a number of ways. One way to classify bone is according to histologic

FIGURE 2-1: HUMAN SKELETON

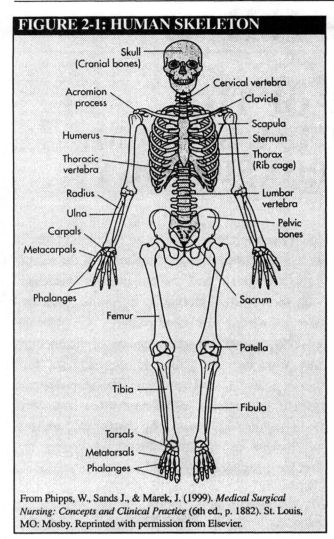

From Phipps, W., Sands J., & Marek, J. (1999). *Medical Surgical Nursing: Concepts and Clinical Practice* (6th ed., p. 1882). St. Louis, MO: Mosby. Reprinted with permission from Elsevier.

structure, as either cancellous or compact. Cancellous bone, or spongy bone, has thin processes and multiple open areas, producing a sponge-like appearance. The bone tissue in cancellous bone contains red and yellow marrow. Compact bone, or dense bone, consists of structural units known as Haversian systems. These systems are arranged in tight proximity to each other, producing a dense bone tissue. The Haversian system serves to transport blood to bone tissue (Ruda, 2000a).

Bone may also be classified according to shape. There are four shapes to bone: flat, irregular, short and long. Flat bones consist of two layers of compact bone with a layer of cancellous bone containing bone marrow sandwiched in the middle. Examples of flat bones include the scapula and skull. Irregular bone comes in different sizes and shapes. The verte-brae are an example of irregular bone. Short bones consist mainly of cancellous bone with a thin covering of compact bone. The bones in the hands and feet are examples of short bones. Long bones have two ends known as epiphyses, and a middle shaft called the diaphysis. Examples of long bones are the femur and the humerus.

Bone Structure

Long bones structurally consist of sections called epiphysis, metaphysis, and diaphysis (see Figure 2-2). The epiphyses, which form the ends of the long bone, are made of cancellous bone. In adults, red bone marrow is found in the epiphyses. The ends of the epiphysis are covered by smooth articular cartilage. The shaft of the long bone is called the diaphysis. The diaphysis consists of compact bone and provides support. The center of the diaphysis contains the medullary cavity, which is filled with yellow bone marrow. In children, the medullary cavity also contains red bone marrow. The area between the epiphysis and diaphysis is the metaphysis. During the years of bone growth, the metaphysis is the location of the epiphyseal growth plate. The epiphyseal growth plate is made of bone-producing cartilage, which allows bones to grow and develop length-wise. Childhood injury of the epiphyseal growth plate, such as a fracture, can impair the continued growth of the bone. Following puberty, the epiphyseal growth plate becomes calcified and ceases bone production. Adults do not have an epiphyseal growth plate (Mourad, 2000).

The long bone is covered by a tough, connective tissue called the periosteum. The periosteum's outer layer contains nerves and blood vessels, some of which penetrate to the inner portion of the bone (Mourad, 2000). A disruption of the periosteum can lead to a separation of the periosteum from the bone and affect the blood supply of that specific area of bone. Osteoblasts, which are bone-forming cells, reside in the periosteum's inner layer (Ruda, 2000a).

FIGURE 2-2: CROSS SECTION OF A LONG BONE

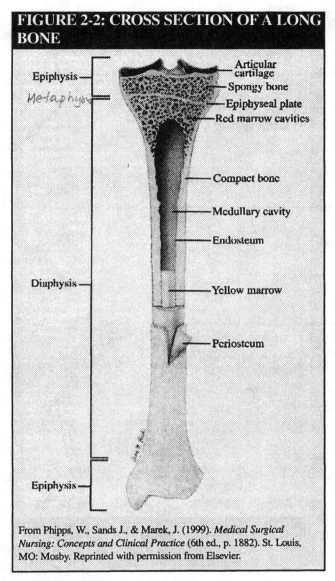

Epiphysis
Metaphysis
Articular cartilage
Spongy bone
Epiphyseal plate
Red marrow cavities
Compact bone
Medullary cavity
Endosteum
Diaphysis
Yellow marrow
Periosteum
Epiphysis

From Phipps, W., Sands J., & Marek, J. (1999). *Medical Surgical Nursing: Concepts and Clinical Practice* (6th ed., p. 1882). St. Louis, MO: Mosby. Reprinted with permission from Elsevier.

Cellular Bone Structure

There are essentially three types of bone cells. *Osteoblasts* are bone-forming cells; and they are necessary for the development of new bone. Osteoblasts eventually become osteocytes. *Osteocytes* are mature bone cells that are present in the bone matrix. *Osteoclasts* are bone-resorbing cells that are responsible for breaking down and resorbing bone (Mourad, 2000). The osteoblasts and osteoclasts are primarily responsible for the process of bone growth and repair.

Osteoblasts and osteoclasts work together to remodel bone, which is the process of developing new bone and removing old bone. When this process maintains its equilibrium, bone integrity,

shape, and strength is preserved. However, there are numerous factors that can disrupt this process, resulting in pathophysiological conditions. Medications, hormone imbalances, genetic predisposition, and poor nutrition are some of the factors that can lead to an imbalance in the remodeling process. Osteoporosis, which develops when osteoclastic activity exceeds osteoblastic activity leading to the development of porous bone, is one example of such a pathological condition.

JOINTS

Function of Joints

Joints occur in the body wherever two bones come together. The formation of joints allows for movement between the bones. Joints are most frequently classified by the amount of movement they permit. Joints may be classified as freely movable (diarthrodial or synovial), slightly movable (amphiarthrotic), or immovable (synarthrotic). The freely movable, or diarthrodial, joints are the most common. There are six types of diarthrodial joints (Ruda, 2000a). See Figure 2–3 for a description of the categories of diarthrodial joints, movement produced, and examples of each joint category.

Structure of Joints

Diarthrodial joints consist of two bone ends that are joined together by connective tissue forming a joint capsule. The joint capsule encloses the bone ends and forms a joint cavity. The end of each bone is covered with articular cartilage that provides a smooth surface for ease of movement between the bones. In addition, the joint capsule is lined by a synovial membrane that secretes synovial fluid, further lubricating the bone ends (Figure 2-4). The combination of articular cartilage and synovial fluid decreases friction between the bones and provides pain-free movement and weight-bearing capability.

FIGURE 2-3: TYPES OF DIARTHRODIAL JOINTS

Joint	Movement	Examples	Illustration
Hinge joint	Flexion, extension	Elbow joint (shown), interphalangeal joints, knee joint	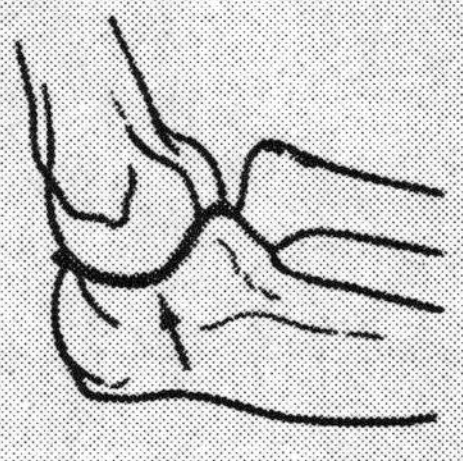
Ball and socket (spheroidal)	Flexion, extension; adduction, abduction; circumduction	Shoulder (shown), hip	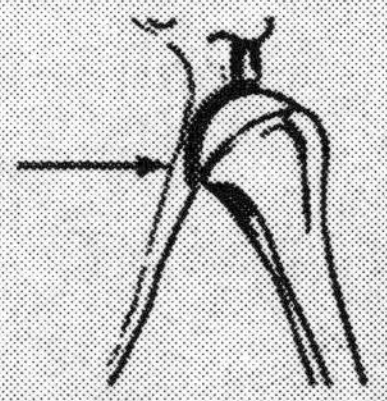
Pivot (rotary)	Rotation	Atlas-axis, proximal radioulnar joint (shown)	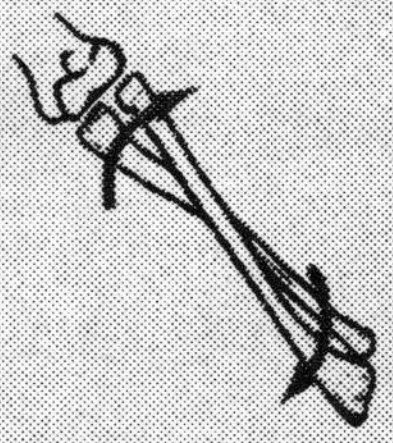
Condyloid	Flexion, extension; abduction, adduction; circumduction	Wrist joint (between radial and carpals) (shown)	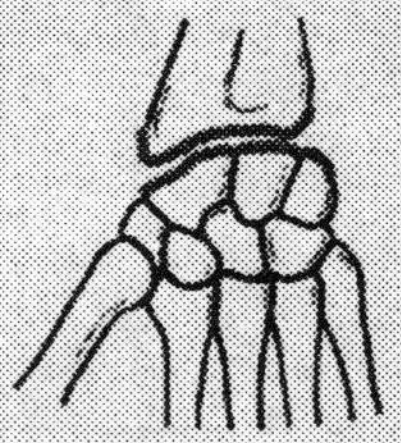
Saddle	Flexion, extension; abduction, adduction; circumduction, thumb-finger opposition	Carpometacarpal joint of thumb	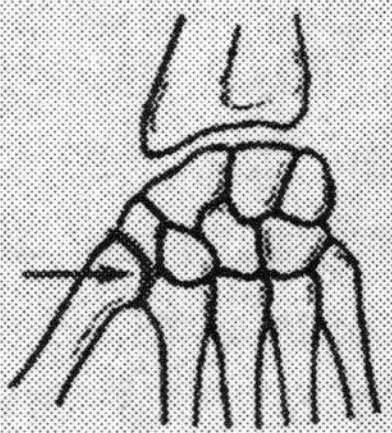
Gliding	One surface moves over another surface	Between tarsal bones, sacroiliac joint, between articular processes of vertebrae, between carpal bones (shown)	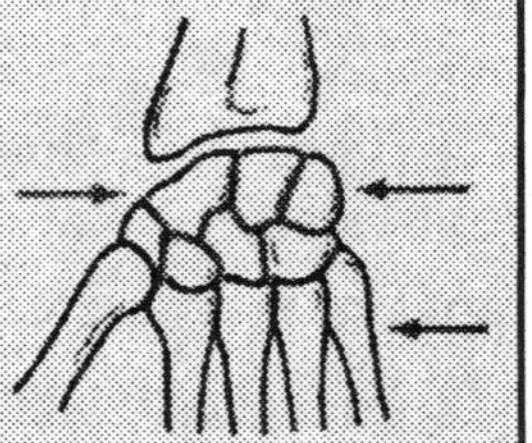

FIGURE 2-4: STRUCTURE OF A SYNOVIAL JOINT

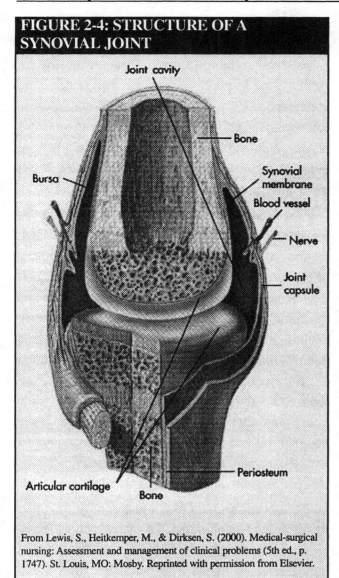

Joint cavity

Bone

Synovial membrane

Blood vessel

Bursa

Nerve

Joint capsule

Periosteum

Articular cartilage

Bone

From Lewis, S., Heitkemper, M., & Dirksen, S. (2000). Medical-surgical nursing: Assessment and management of clinical problems (5th ed., p. 1747). St. Louis, MO: Mosby. Reprinted with permission from Elsevier.

CARTILAGE

Function and Structure of Cartilage

Cartilage is a connective tissue that forms a protective covering and provides support for the structures that lie underneath. As mentioned previously, cartilage plays an important role in creating a smooth surface between bone ends to facilitate joint movement in diarthrodial joints. Cartilage cells reproduce slowly and are slow to heal if damaged (Ruda, 2000a).

LIGAMENTS AND TENDONS

Function and Structure of Ligaments and Tendons

Ligaments and tendons are made of a fibrous connective tissue known as collagen. Ligaments provide joint stability by connecting joints together and preventing excessive movement within the joints. Tendons actually attach muscle to bone (Ruda, 2000a).

SKELETAL MUSCLES

Function of Skeletal Muscle

There are three types of muscle tissue in the human body — cardiac, smooth, and skeletal. Cardiac muscle and smooth muscle produce involuntary movement and will not be addressed in this discussion. Skeletal muscle, which is the largest muscle mass in the body, produces voluntary movement as a result of neuronal stimulation. The function of skeletal muscle is to produce movement and support posture through the process of muscle contractions (Ruda, 2000a).

Structure of Skeletal Muscle

Skeletal muscles are composed of muscle fibers (cells). Each muscle fiber contains myofibrils that are capable of contracting due to the presence of numerous thick and thin filaments of contractile protein. The thick filaments are composed of myosin protein, and the thin filaments are composed of actin protein. Together these two types of filaments make up the sarcomere, which is the myofibril's contractile unit. When the myosin filaments and actin filaments slide past each other, the sarcomere is shortened, and a muscle contraction is produced (Ruda, 2000a).

For muscle contractions to occur, neuronal stimulation must be present at the muscle cell. Nerve fibers come in contact with muscle cells at the neuromuscular junction. When acetylcholine is released at the neuromuscular junction by the nerve fiber, it diffuses across the neuromuscular junction to stimulate the receptors of the muscle fiber. Calcium ions are released from the muscle fiber, causing contraction in the myofibrils. In addition to neuronal stimulation, muscle contraction also requires an energy source. Adenosine triphosphate (ATP) and creatine phosphate provide this energy source (Ruda, 2000a).

There are two types of muscle contractions — isometric and isotonic. In isometric muscle contractions, the muscle tension increases while the length of the muscle remains the same. No movement is produced. An example of an isometric contraction would be the increased tension that is produced by pressing the hand and arm against an immovable object such as a wall. In an isotonic contraction, the muscle tension stays the same but the length of the muscle changes. Lifting weights are an example of the type of activity accomplished through an isotonic contraction (Mourad, 2000).

MUSCULOSKELETAL SYSTEM AND THE AGING PROCESS

It is important for nurses to understand the changes that occur in the musculoskeletal system as a result of the aging process. As the percentage of elderly in the United States population continues to increase, nurses will care for more and more elderly patients who are experiencing health problems of the musculoskeletal system and altered functioning as a result. Nurse's must remain aware that altered activity levels and impaired mobility can rapidly impact the functioning of the musculoskeletal system, even in previously healthy individuals.

One of the most significant changes that occurs is in the bone remodeling process. The osteoblastic activity of the bones begins to decrease, with less new bone being developed, while osteoclastic activ-

ity increases. This alteration in the bone remodeling process results in more bone being reabsorbed and a decrease in bone density. Osteoporosis is the potential end result, leaving the individual at an increased risk for bone fractures (Ruda, 2000a). Encouraging individuals to maintain an adequate intake of calcium and a program of weight-bearing exercise to prevent bone loss are important health promotion activities for the nurse.

As aging occurs, changes also develop in the muscles, joints, tendons, and ligaments. Cartilage begins to calcify, affecting joint movement. Mobility is also affected as the joints, tendons, and ligaments become less flexible. Muscle mass begins to shrink, affecting muscle strength. Neuronal stimulation of the muscles is slowed, increasing reaction time (Ruda, 2000a). The nurse should encourage health promotion activities that preserve function such as a walking exercise program, flexibility exercises, and activities that promote full and active range of motion. The nurse should also encourage a well-balanced diet that will help maintain a desired weight, thus preventing excess stress on the joints.

It is not inevitable that aging lead to impaired mobility and functioning. By incorporating health promotion activities for the musculoskeletal system into their daily lifestyle, individuals can decrease the effects of aging and maintain a desirable level of functioning.

SUMMARY

To best understand musculoskeletal diseases and disorders and the nursing care associated with these health problems, the orthopedic nurse must be knowledgeable about the anatomy and physiology of the musculoskeletal system. This chapter provided an overview of the structures of the musculoskeletal system and the basic physiologic processes that govern bone growth and repair. As many of the patients who experience musculoskeletal problems are elderly, the chapter also addressed how the aging process affects the normal physiological processes occurring within the bones, muscles, and other structures of the musculoskeletal system. This foundation supplies the nurse with the knowledge necessary to provide quality nursing care.

EXAM QUESTIONS

CHAPTER 2
Questions 5–13

5. One function of bone is to

   a. produce voluntary movement.

   b. provide structural support

   c. promote joint stability.

   d. maintain upright posture.

6. Injury to the epiphyseal growth plate during childhood can result in

   a. osteoarthritis.

   b. impaired bone growth.

   c. chronic joint pain.

   d. decreased bone mass.

7. Bone-forming cells are called

   a. osteoblasts.

   b. osteoclasts.

   c. osteocytes.

   d. ossifications.

8. An imbalance in the bone remodeling process can result from

   a. adolescent growth spurts.

   b. excessive weight bearing exercise.

   c. excessive Vitamin C intake.

   d. hormone imbalances.

9. Joints that are freely movable are classified as

   a. synarthrotic joints.

   b. amphiarthrotic joints.

   c. diarthrodial joints.

   d. articular joints.

10. The function of articular cartilage is to

    a. provide a smooth surface between bone ends.

    b. connect muscle to bone.

    c. secrete synovial fluid.

    d. increase joint range of motion.

11. Structures that provide joint stability are called

    a. tendons.

    b. skeletal muscle.

    c. cartilage.

    d. ligaments.

12. One of the functions of skeletal muscle is to

    a. support posture.

    b. protect bone.

    c. connect joints.

    d. prevent excessive joint movement.

13. As a result of the aging process, changes in the musculoskeletal system include

    a. softening of joint cartilage.

    b. increased ligament flexibility.

    c. shortening of the long bones.

    d. decreased osteoblastic activity.

CHAPTER 3

NURSING ASSESSMENT OF PATIENTS WITH MUSCULOSKELETAL DISORDERS

CHAPTER OBJECTIVE

After completing this chapter, the reader will be able to describe how to perform an assessment of the musculoskeletal system.

LEARNING OBJECTIVES

After studying this chapter, the reader will be able to

1. indicate the subjective data that is gathered when performing an assessment of the musculoskeletal system.

2. specify the physical assessment techniques that are appropriate when performing an assessment of the musculoskeletal system.

3. differentiate the normal and abnormal findings that may be noted during the physical assessment of the musculoskeletal system.

OVERVIEW

Nurse's in orthopedic practice are responsible for assessing patients to identify potential or actual health problems related to the musculoskeletal system. These health problems are related to structural abnormalities and/or impaired function. A musculoskeletal assessment consists of two parts: the nursing history and the physical assessment. This chapter will describe the subjective data that is gathered from the patient during the nursing history and the objective data that the nurse gathers when performing a physical assessment of the musculoskeletal system. The chapter also describes the normal findings of a musculoskeletal assessment, as well as potentially abnormal findings.

NURSING HISTORY

The nurse begins any initial patient assessment by conducting a nursing history. The purpose of the nursing history is to gather subjective data about the patient's chief complaint and concerns, past medical history, activities of daily living, functional ability, and mobility. It is also important to gather information about the patient's socioeconomic status, cultural beliefs and values, health beliefs, and the patient's desired outcome for any medical or nursing interventions. The nurse should also assess the patient's readiness and ability to learn. Data related to the patient's educational background, preferred learning styles, and ability to comprehend new information can be meaningful in the development of a patient education plan. The nurse will use the data gathered in the nursing history to establish an individualized plan of care for the patient.

The extent of the nursing history will depend upon the nature of the patient's health problem. For example, if the patient has experienced a traumatic accident and is in acute pain, the nurse will concentrate on gathering the data most crucial to providing safe, immediate care to the patient and defer the remainder of the nursing history to a more appropriate time. Also, some musculoskeletal system problems are more localized (i.e., sprained ankle) while other problems, such as joint pain related to rheumatoid arthritis, are more systemic. The nurse should conduct a nursing history that is appropriate to the nature of the health problem.

Chief Complaint

The nurse starts the nursing history by asking the patient for information about the chief problem or symptom that lead him or her to seek health care. Some common symptoms for which individuals with musculoskeletal problems seek health care include: joint or muscle pain; alteration in muscle strength, gait, joint movement, or function; change in appearance; swelling; and sensory changes such as paresthesia. After determining what the chief complaint is, the nurse should ask additional questions about onset and duration of the symptom, precipitating factors, alleviating factors, and how the symptom has affected the performance of the individual's daily activities.

Past Medical History

The nurse should review the patient's past medical history to identify any previous history of musculoskeletal disorders or predisposing factors that can lead to the development of a musculoskeletal problem. In addition, the nurse will want to gather information about any co-existing health problems such as cardiovascular disease, chronic respiratory disorders, or diabetes, as these conditions can be adversely affected by immobility and alterations in daily living activities. Chronic health problems can also interfere with the treatment of musculoskeletal disorders or the healing process. Lifestyle choices such as use of tobacco, drugs, and alcohol should also be assessed, as they can contribute to chronic health problems.

Review of Systems

During the nursing history, the nurse will want to conduct a review of systems to gather data that will help develop a plan of care for the patient. Areas of special concern include nutrition, activity, exercise and rest, elimination, and psychosocial issues.

Nutrition

Adequate nutrition is important to maintaining strong bones and muscles. Specifically the nurse should assess for adequate intake of foods containing calcium, vitamin D, vitamin C, and protein (Ruda, 2000a). The use of vitamin and calcium supplements should also be noted. Any recent weight loss or gain is documented. A determination of the patient's ideal weight should also be calculated. Obesity can cause stress in weight-bearing joints, increase pain, and decrease mobility, so maintenance of a normal weight is encouraged.

Activity, Exercise, and Rest

The patient should be asked to describe his or her normal activities of daily living and any difficulties that exist in performing these activities. For example, arthritis can make such simple activities as dressing oneself, combing hair, using the toilet, and tying shoestrings difficult to perform without assistance. Opening jars and preparing food can also become difficult with stiff and painful finger joints. Walking up and down stairs or on uneven surfaces can also become difficult or dangerous to attempt. The nurse should also ask how the patient is compensating for any difficulties that have developed and determine if special equipment/assistive devices are needed to help promote mobility or the performance of other activities.

The nurse should also inquire if the patient has a regular exercise routine and about any activity requirements related to employment. Some jobs may require much walking and heavy lifting, while other jobs are sedentary in nature but put the patient at risk of repetitive motion injuries. The patient should be asked how exercise and the performance of job-related activities are affected by the musculoskeletal problem.

Another area that needs exploration is the patient's sleeping pattern. The nurse should ask the patient how many hours of sleep are obtained nightly and if sleep is interrupted by pain or the need for frequent changes of position.

Elimination

The most common elimination problem associated with musculoskeletal disorders is constipation related to immobility. In addition, some musculoskeletal disorders can lead to functional bowel and bladder incontinence (Ruda, 2000a). The nurse should gather data about the patient's bowel and bladder elimination patterns and any difficulties that the patient may have with using toilet facilities independently. The use of assistive devices such as toilet extenders and grab bars should also be addressed.

Psychosocial Issues

Musculoskeletal disorders can affect the patient's psychosocial status in a number of different ways. First of all, the patient may experience difficulty with stress and ineffective coping related to the development of an acute or chronic health problem that affects mobility, causes pain, and leads to a lack of independence. The nurse should question the patient about usual coping mechanisms and ask how the patient is coping with the current health care problem. The patient's roles and responsibilities as a spouse, parent, friend, and/or employee can also be altered by the development of a musculoskeletal problem. Pain and discomfort may interfere with sexual relationships. The development of a chronic disability or deformity can lead to body image changes and an altered self-concept. In addition, a chronic illness or an extended recovery from an acute musculoskeletal disorder can have serious financial implications for the patient. The nurse should carefully gather data related to all of these areas to determine how the patient is coping with the health problem.

Assessment of Cultural Background

A patient's cultural background will affect how the patient will respond to treatment. Likewise, the nurse's cultural background will affect his or her response to patients. It is important that nurse's assess the patient's cultural beliefs and values so that nursing care can be delivered in a culturally sensitive manner. It is also essential that nurses examine their own personal beliefs and biases and acknowledge that these views can affect the nursing care they provide their clients. Being aware of one's beliefs and biases can help the nurse avoid ethnocentrism, which is the belief that one's own culture is better than another (Kotch, 2001). There are many books on providing culturally competent nursing care that can provide the nurse with insight into the beliefs of different cultures.

The first step to providing culturally sensitive health care is to perform a cultural assessment. The major components of a cultural assessment include gathering data related to the patient's beliefs about health, illness, and health care, religious practices, and food preferences. The patient should be asked about any specific health care practices that are meaningful to him or her. The meaning of pain in the person's culture and how the person copes with pain is a particularly significant assessment for the nurse to make. The family social structure should be assessed as well as communication patterns. The concepts of time, territoriality, and personal space are other important factors to consider. The nurse should interview the patient in a respectful manner and explain that the information will be used to provide nursing care that respects the patient's beliefs.

Assessment of Pain

Pain is frequently the chief complaint that leads a patient to seek out health care for a musculoskeletal disorder. The nurse should carefully inquire about the conditions under which the pain occur:

- Does pain occur only upon movement or weight-bearing activities, or does it also occur when the affected body part is at rest?

- Is the pain localized to one joint or body part, or is the pain more systemic in nature?

- Does the pain radiate?

- Is the pain affecting the patient's ability to sleep at night?

- Is the pain accompanied by any other symptoms such as swelling, inflammation, loss of function, or obvious deformity?

- Is there any altered sensation in the affected body part, such as numbness, tingling, or burning sensations?

The patient should be asked to describe the pain, including type and severity of pain, location, duration, precipitating factors, and what the patient does to relieve pain (Schoen, 2000). A numeric pain scale or visual analog scale (Figure 3-1) is the most accurate means of rating the severity of a patient's pain. By using a pain scale to rate pain, the nurse can more easily assess the effectiveness of any treatment.

Medications that Adversely Affect the Musculoskeletal System

The nurse should carefully question the patient about any medications that he or she may be taking. There are a number of commonly prescribed medications that can adversely affect the musculoskeletal system. For example, long-term use of corticosteroids can lead to the development of osteoporosis and muscle weakness. Antiseizure medications can cause osteomalacia. Phenothiazines can affect the patient's gait. Diuretics that deplete serum potassium levels can cause muscle weakness and cramps (Ruda, 2000a).

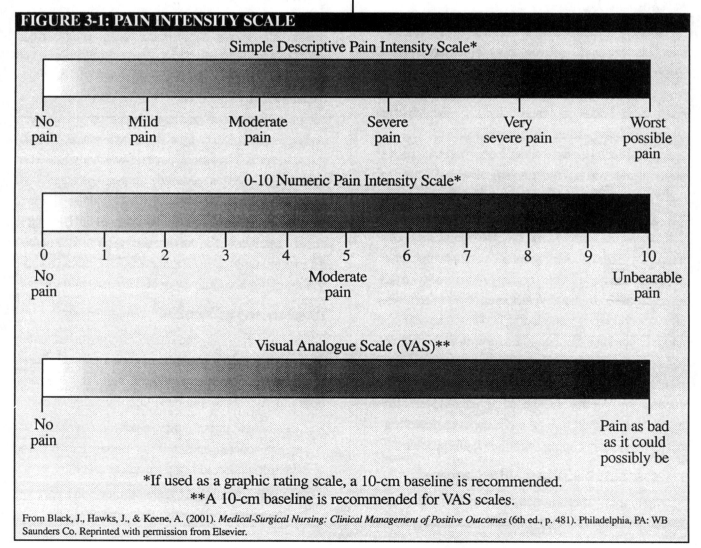

FIGURE 3-1: PAIN INTENSITY SCALE

Simple Descriptive Pain Intensity Scale*

No pain | Mild pain | Moderate pain | Severe pain | Very severe pain | Worst possible pain

0-10 Numeric Pain Intensity Scale*

0 1 2 3 4 5 6 7 8 9 10

No pain | Moderate pain | Unbearable pain

Visual Analogue Scale (VAS)**

No pain | Pain as bad as it could possibly be

*If used as a graphic rating scale, a 10-cm baseline is recommended.
**A 10-cm baseline is recommended for VAS scales.

From Black, J., Hawks, J., & Keene, A. (2001). *Medical-Surgical Nursing: Clinical Management of Positive Outcomes* (6th ed., p. 481). Philadelphia, PA: WB Saunders Co. Reprinted with permission from Elsevier.

PHYSICAL ASSESSMENT

Following completion of the nursing history, the nurse will gather objective data by conducting a systematic physical assessment. The techniques of inspection and palpation are the primary methods by which nurses conduct the physical assessment of the musculoskeletal system. The nurse will assess the patient's posture, gait, joint range of motion, muscle mass, muscle strength, and neurovascular status (Liddel, 2000a). All normal and abnormal findings are documented. Common abnormalities of the musculoskeletal system that the nurse may observe can be found in Table 3-1.

Assessment of Posture and Gait

The nurse inspects the patient's sitting and standing posture as well as gait. This assessment can begin with the initial patient contact as the nurse observes the individual's unconscious, natural movements (Schoen, 2000). The nurse can also ask the patient to walk across the room to assess gait and posture more deliberately. The gait should have a smooth rhythm with steady, well-balanced movements. Normally the length of stride is approximately 15 inches, with the heels about 2-4 inches apart from each other as the patient walks. The arms normally swing freely in rhythm with the stride. Posture is erect (Casteel, 2003; Schoen, 2000).

To adequately assess the patient's posture, the entire length of the spine, buttocks, and legs should be exposed for inspection (Liddel, 2000a). The nurse closely examines the spinal alignment, both laterally and posteriorly, with the patient standing to detect any abnormal curvatures and deformities. Normally, the spine will be convex in the thoracic area and concave in the cervical and lumbar areas. The height of the shoulders and iliac crests should be symmetrical. Gluteal folds should also be symmetric. The nurse also asks the patient to bend forward to detect any spinal curvature or rising scapula.

Some common abnormalities that might be detected in the spine are scoliosis, lordosis, and kyphosis (Liddel, 2000a). Scoliosis, a lateral curvature of the spine, commonly develops in adolescents. Lordosis (swayback) is an exaggeration of the concave curvature of the lumbar area. Kyphosis is an exaggeration of the convex curvature of the thoracic spine. Kyphosis results in a rounded back that is frequently associated with the development of osteoporosis and the collapse of thoracic vertebrae.

Any abnormalities noted by the nurse are documented.

Assessment of Joint Movement

Assessment of joint movement and range of motion is another important component of the examination of the musculoskeletal system. The nurse should inspect and palpate the joint for any evidence of abnormal positioning, deformity, or swelling before putting the joint through any range of motion exercises. Range of motion is classified as active or passive. Active range of motion is performed by the patient without any assistance from others. With passive range of motion, the nurse moves the joint through the range of motion for the patient. When performing passive range of motion, the nurse should be careful not to move the joint past the point of pain or resistance, or damage to the joint may occur. Each joint should be completely exposed during examination and range of motion. A goniometer is used to accurately measure the range of motion of each joint when a limitation of movement is detected (Ruda, 2000a).

Any joint movement limitations or deformities are documented. Limitations to joint movement are frequently due to the development of contractures or to dislocations or subluxation of the joint. In addition to any limitation of joint movement, the nurse should also palpate the joint for effusion and any crepitus during movement. Crepitus is a grating or crackling sound in the joint that can be felt or heard; it indicates that the joint surfaces are no longer smoothly articulating, most likely due to degenerative joint disease (Liddel, 2000a). The

TABLE 3-1: ASSESSMENT ABNORMALITIES OF THE MUSCULOSKELETAL SYSTEM

Finding	Description	Possible Etiology and Significance
Ankylosis	Scarring within a joint leading to stiffness or fixation	Chronic joint inflammation
Atrophy	Wasting of muscle, characterized by decrease in circumference and flabby appearance and resulting in decrease in function and muscle tone	Prolonged disuse, contracture, immobilization, muscle denervation
Contracture	Resistance to movement of muscle or joint as result of fibrosis or supporting soft tissues	Shortening of muscle or ligament structure, tightness of soft tissue, immobilization, incorrect positioning
Crepitation	Crackling sound or grating sensation as result of friction between bones	Fracture, chronic inflammation, dislocation
Effusion	Fluid in joint possible with swelling and pain	Trauma, especially to knee
Felon	Abscess occurring in pulp space (tissue mass) of distal phalanx of finger as a result of infection	Minor hand injury, puncture wound, laceration
Ganglion	Small, fluid-filled synovial cyst usually on dorsal surface of wrist and foot	Degeneration of connective tissue close to tendons and joints leading to formation of small cysts
Hypertrophy	Increase in size of muscle as result of enlargement of existing cells	Exercise, increased androgens, increased stimulation or use
Kyphosis (round back)	Anteroposterior or forward bending of spine with convexity of curve in posterior direction; common at thoracic and sacral levels	Poor posture, tuberculosis, chronic arthritis, growth disturbance of vertebral epiphysis, osteoporosis
Lordosis	Deformity of spine resulting in anteroposterior curvature with concavity in posterior direction; common in lumbar spine	Secondary to other deformities of spine, muscular dystrophy, obesity, flexion contracture of hip, congenital dislocation of hip
Pes planus	Flatfoot	Congenital condition, muscle paralysis, mild cerebral palsy, early muscular dystrophy
Scoliosis	Deformity resulting in lateral curvature of spine	Idiopathic or congenital condition, fracture or dislocation, osteomalacia, functional condition
Subluxation	Partial dislocation of joint	Instability of joint capsule and supporting ligaments (e.g., from trauma, arthritis)
Valgus	Angulation of bone away from midline	Alteration in gait, pain, abnormal erosion of articular cartilage
Varus	Angulation of bone toward midline	Alteration in gait, pain, abnormal erosion of articular cartilage

From Lewis, S., Heitkemper, M., & Dirksen, S. (2000). *Medical-surgical nursing: Assessment and management of clinical problems* (5th ed., p. 1755). St. Louis, MO: Mosby. Reprinted with permission from Elsevier.

nurse should also assess the joint for heat, pain, or tenderness (Casteel, 2003).

A description of movements that can occur with synovial joints is listed in Table 3-2. A complete listing of the normal range of motion for each joint can be found illustrated in Table 3-3.

Assessment of Muscle Mass and Strength

Muscle mass is assessed by measuring the circumference of the muscle with a tape measure. Muscles are measured bilaterally at the maximum circumference of the muscle. The muscles should be resting in the same position when measured. If repeated measures are to be taken, it is appropriate to place a marking on the skin at the location of the measurement so that future measurements will be taken at the same location. The muscle size of the unaffected extremity is compared to the affected extremity. Either muscle swelling or muscle atrophy can be detected in this manner. Some differences in muscle size are normal and to be anticipated. Any differences in size greater than 1 centimeter are considered to be significant (Liddel, 2000a).

Muscle strength can be assessed during the examination of range of motion by having the patient pull or press against any restrictions applied by the nurse. The nurse makes a comparison of bilateral muscle strength, keeping in mind that the dominant arm and leg will typically demonstrate more strength (Schoen, 2000).

Neurovascular Status

Because many musculoskeletal injuries can cause nerve or blood vessel damage, it is important to include an assessment of the neurovascular status of the involved extremities (Kunkler, 1999). When assessing the neurovascular status, the nurse carefully notes the circulation, motion, and sensation of the involved extremity, and promptly reports any abnormal findings. A delay in reporting an impaired neurovascular status can quickly lead to permanent neuromuscular damage and loss of function.

Circulation is assessed by noting quality of pulses, any swelling, the color and temperature of the extremity, and by checking capillary refill (Altizer, 2002). The assessment findings are compared to the unaffected extremity to note any differences. The nurse should promptly report any findings that suggest circulatory compromise: edema, decreased pulses or pulselessness, cool temperature of the extremity, pale color, and capillary refill of greater than 3 seconds.

TABLE 3-2: MOVEMENT AT SYNOVIAL JOINTS

Movement	Description
Flexion	Bending of joint that decreases angle between two boines; shortening of muscle length
Extension	Bending of joint that increases angle between two bones
Hyperextension	Extension in which angle exceeds 180 degrees
Abduction	Movement of part away from midline
Adduction	Movement of part toward midline
Pronation	Turning of palm downward or sole outward
Supination	Turning of palm upward or sole inward
Circumduction	Combination of flexion, extension, abduction, and adduction resulting in circular motion of body part
Rotation	Movement about longitudinal axis
Inversion	Turnign of sole inward toward midline
Eversion	Turning of sole outward away from midline

From Lewis, S., Heitkemper, M., & Dirksen, S. (2000). *Medical-surgical nursing: Assessment and management of clinical problems* (5th ed., p. 1754). St. Louis, MO: Mosby. Reprinted with permission from Elsevier.

TABLE 3-3: RANGE OF MOTION EXERCISES

Body Part	Type of Joint	Type of Movement	Range (Degrees)	Primary Muscles
Neck, cervical spine	Pivotal	*Flexion:* Bring chin to rest on chest	45	Sternocleidomastoid
		Extension: Bend head back as far as possible	10	Trapezius
		Lateral flexion: Tilt head as far as possible toward each shoulder	40-45	Sternocleidomastoid
		Rotation: Tilt head as far as possible in circular movement	180	Sternocleidomastoid trapezius
Shoulder	Ball and socket	*Flexion:* Raise arm from side position forward to position above head	170-180	Coracobrachialis, deltoid,
		Extension: Move arm behind body, keeping elbow straight	45-60	Latissimus dorsi, teres major, deltoid
		Abduction: Raise arm to side to position above head with palm away from head	170-180	Deltoid, supraspinatus Pectoralis major
		Adduction: Lower arm sideways and across body as far as possible		
		Internal rotation: With elbow flexed, rotate shoulder by moving arm until thumb is turned inward and toward back.	70-80	Pectoralis major, latissimus dorsi, teres major, subscapularis
		External rotation: With elbow in full circle, move arm until thumb is upward and lateral to head	81-90	Infraspinatus, teres major

TABLE 3-3: RANGE OF MOTION EXERCISES (CONTINUED)

Body Part	Type of Joint	Type of Movement	Range (Degrees)	Primary Muscles
Shoulder, cont'd		*Circumduction:* Move arm in full circle (Circumduction is combination of all movements of ball-and-socket joint.)	360	Deltoid, coracobrachialis, latissimus dorsi, teres major
Elbow	Hinge	*Flexion:* Bend elbow so that lower arm moves toward its shoulder joint and hand is level with shoulder.	150	Biceps brachii, brachialis, brachio-radialis
		Extension: Straighten elbow by lowering hand	150	Triceps brachii
Forearm	Pivotal	*Supination:* Turn lower arm and hand so that palm is up	70-90	Supinator, biceps brachii
		Pronation: Turn lower arm so that palm is down	70-90	Pronator teres, pronator quadratus
Wrist	Condyloid	*Flexion:* Move palm toward inner aspect of forearm	80-90	Flexor carpi ulnaris, flexor carpi radialis
		Extension: Bring dorsal surface of hand back as far as possible	89-90	Extensor carpi radialis brevis, extensor carpi radialis longus, extensor carpi ulnaris
		Abduction (radial deviation): Bend wrist medially toward thumb	Up to 30	Flexor carpi radialis, extensor carpi radialis brevis, extensor carpi radialis longus
		Adduction (ulnar deviation): Bend wrist laterally toward fifth finger	30-50	Flexor carpi ulnaris, extensor carpi ulnaris

TABLE 3-3: RANGE OF MOTION EXERCISES (CONTINUED)

Body Part	Type of Joint	Type of Movement	Range (Degrees)	Primary Muscles
Fingers	Condyloid hinge	*Flexion:* Make fist	90	Lumbricales, interosseus volaris, interosseus dorsalis
		Extension: Bend fingers back as far as possible	30-60	Extensor digiti quinti proprius, extensor digitorum communis, extensor indicis proprius
		Abduction: Spread fingers apart	30	Interosseus dorsalis
		Adduction: Bring fingers together	30	Interosseus volaris
Thumb	Saddle	*Flexion:* Move thumb across palmar surface of hand		Flexor pollicis brevis
		Extension: Move thumb straight away from hand		Extensor pollicis longus, extensor pollicis brevis
		Abduction: Extend thumb laterally (usually done when placing fingers in abduction and adduction)	70-80	Abductor pollicis brevis and longus
		Adduction: Move thumb back toward hand	70-80	Adductor pollicis obliquus, adductor pollicis transversus
		Opposition: Touch thumb to each finger of		Opponeus pollicis, opponeus digiti minimi
Hip	Ball and socket	*Flexion:* Move leg forward and up	120-130	Psoas major, iliacus, sartorius
		Extension: Move back beside other leg	120-130	Gluteus maximus, semitendinodud, semimembranosus

TABLE 3-3: RANGE OF MOTION EXERCISES (CONTINUED)

Body Part	Type of Joint	Type of Movement	Range (Degrees)	Primary Muscles
Hip cont'd		*Hyperextension:* Move leg behind body	10-20	Gluteus maximus, semitendinosus, semimembranosus
		Abduction: Move leg laterally away from body	30-50	Gluteus medius, gluteus minimus
		Adduction: Move leg back toward medial position and beyond if possible	20-30	Adductor longus, adductor brevis, adductor magnus
		Internal rotation: Turn foot and leg toward other leg	35-45	Gluteus medius, gluteus minimus tensor fasciae latae
		External rotation: Turn foot and leg away from other leg	40-50	Obturatorius internus, obutratorius externus, quadratus femoris, piriformis, gemellus superior and inferior, gluteus maximus
		Circumduction: Move leg in circle		Psoas major, gluteus maximus, gluteus medius, adductor magnus
Knee	Hinge	*Flexion:* Bring heel back toward back of thigh	135-145	Biceps femoris, semitendinosus, semimembranosus, sartorius
		Extension: Return leg to floor	0	Rectus femoris, vastus lateralis, vastus medialis, vastus intermedius

TABLE 3-3: RANGE OF MOTION EXERCISES (CONTINUED)

Body Part	Type of Joint	Type of Movement	Range (Degrees)	Primary Muscles
Ankle	Hinge	*Dorsal flexion:* Move foot so that toes are pointed upward	20-30	Tibialis anterior
		Plantar flexion: Move foot so that toes are pointed downward	45-50	Gastrocnemius, soleus
Foot	Gliding	*Inversion:* Turn sole of foot medially	30-40	Tibialis anterior, tibialis posterior
		Eversion: Turn sole of foot laterally	15-25	Peroneus longus, peroneus brevis
Toes	Condyloid	*Flexion:* Curl toes downward	30-60	Flexor digitorum, lumbricalis pedis, flexor hallucis brevis
		Extension: Straighten toes	30-60	Extensor digitorum longus, extensor digitorum brevis, extensor hallucis longus
		Abduction: Spread toes apart	15 or less	Abductor hallucis, interosseus dorsalis
		Adduction: Bring toes together	15 or less	Adductor hallucis, interosseus plantaris

From Potter, P. & Perry, A. (2001). *Fundamentals of nursing* (5th ed., pp. 1501-1505). St. Louis, MO: Mosby. Reprinted with permission from Elsevier.

The neurological status is assessed by checking motion of the affected extremity. Any weakness or paralysis should promptly be reported. In addition, the patient should be questioned about any sensation of paresthesia (tingling), loss of feeling, increasing or unrelieved pain, or pain upon passive stretching of the extremity. Table 3-4 illustrates assessment of peripheral nerves.

SUMMARY

This chapter described the subjective data that is gathered during the nursing history and the objective data that the nurse gathers during the physical assessment of the musculoskeletal system. The chapter also described the normal findings of a musculoskeletal assessment, as well as potentially abnormal findings. It is important that the orthopedic nurse develop sharp assessment skills in order to promptly identify potentially significant changes in the patient's condition. It is also important that the nurse not dismiss even seemingly minor changes in the patient's condition. Failure of the nurse to intervene promptly when complications develop can lead to significant impairment and disability.

TABLE 3-4: PERIPHERAL NERVE FUNCTION ASSESSMENT

Peripheral Nerve	Sensation Test	Movement Test
Median	Prick distal surface or tip of index finger	Have patient flex wrist and oppose thumb to little finger
Radial	Prick skin area between thumb and index finger	Have patient extend fingers, thumb and wrist
Ulnar	Prick top of little finger	Have patient extend and spread fingers
Tibial	Prick sole of foot laterally and medially	Have patient plantar flex foot
Peroneal	Prick skin between great toe and second toe	Have patient dorsiflex foot

EXAM QUESTIONS

CHAPTER 3
Questions 14-20

14. The nurse begins the initial assessment of a patient with a musculoskeletal disorder by

    a. observing the patient's gait.

    b. assessing the patient's muscle strength.

    c. palpating the patient's joints.

    d. conducting a nursing history.

15. Subjective data that the nurse gathers during an assessment of the musculoskeletal system includes the patient's

    a. functional ability.

    b. joint range of motion.

    c. neurovascular status.

    d. spinal alignment.

16. One of the most common chief complaints that leads a patient with a musculoskeletal disorder to seek health care is

    a. joint stiffness.

    b. deformity.

    c. pain.

    d. weak hand grip.

17. The primary methods of assessment that the nurse uses during the physical assessment of the musculoskeletal system are

    a. inspection and palpation.

    b. percussion and palpation.

    c. auscultation and inspection.

    d. auscultation and percussion.

18. During an assessment of the patient's posture, the nurse would normally expect to find

    a. asymmetrical gluteal folds.

    b. convex curvature of the cervical area.

    c. concave curvature of the thoracic area.

    d. symmetrical height of the iliac crests.

19. When performing passive range of motion the nurse should be careful to avoid

    a. exposing the joint and causing the patient to chill.

    b. moving the joint past the point of pain or resistance.

    c. fatiguing the muscle in the extremity being exercised.

    d. distracting the patient with conversation.

20. When crepitus is heard during joint movement it indicates that

    a. there is friction between the bones.

    b. ligaments have lost flexibility.

    c. muscles have developed disuse atrophy.

    d. the patient is elderly and not mobile.

CHAPTER 4

CLINICAL MANIFESTATIONS OF MUSCULOSKELETAL DISORDERS

CHAPTER OBJECTIVE

After completing this chapter, the reader will be able to describe the clinical manifestations of musculoskeletal disorders.

LEARNING OBJECTIVES

After studying this chapter, the reader will be able to

1. identify the common clinical manifestations associated with musculoskeletal disorders.

2. select nursing assessments related to musculoskeletal pain, loss of mobility, and loss of function.

3. indicate nursing interventions related to musculoskeletal pain, loss of mobility, and loss of function.

OVERVIEW

Since the main function of the musculoskeletal system is to provide the structure and support through which our body can produce voluntary, coordinated movements, it stands to reason that a disruption in the system is likely to cause the patient to experience difficulty with mobility and/or functional abilities. This difficulty is frequently accompanied by pain. The orthopedic nurse must understand the common clinical manifestations associated with musculoskeletal disorders and the associated nursing assessments and nursing interventions. This chapter describes the common clinical manifestations of musculoskeletal disorders, which include loss of function, loss of mobility, and musculoskeletal pain. The nursing assessments and nursing interventions associated with these clinical problems are also addressed.

LOSS OF MOBILITY AND FUNCTION

Musculoskeletal disorders can lead to a loss of mobility due to a change in muscle strength, joint range of motion, or function (Eggenberger, 1998). The musculoskeletal system is adversely affected by immobility. Whenever a body part is immobilized, whether by trauma or by some form of immobilization device such as a cast, the muscles and joints quickly begin to lose strength and function from disuse. The potential side effects of immobility, even if just one area of the body is affected, are muscle atrophy, joint instability, limited range of motion, and pressure sores. It takes as little as 4 days of immobility for significant muscle atrophy to begin to develop, even in individuals who were previously healthy (Jagmin, 1998). When caring for a patient with a musculoskeletal disorder, the nurse must always be cognizant of the adverse effects immobility can have on the total body. A careful assessment of the patient's mobility and functional ability must be made on an ongoing basis.

The nurse's initial assessment of any patient with a musculoskeletal disorder should include an assessment of how the disorder is affecting the patient's ability to move and perform self-care activities. The nurse should observe the patient's appearance and note if there is any evidence of poor hygiene, which may be a result of an inability to provide self-care due to a loss of mobility or function. Table 4–1 provides a list of potential nursing diagnoses that are appropriate for patients who have experienced a loss of mobility or function. The orthopedic nurse should anticipate that any patient who has experienced a loss of mobility or function can develop these problems, regardless of age or previous health status. All patients should be carefully assessed accordingly, and nursing interventions should be implemented to prevent the development of these problems. Table 4–2 identifies nursing interventions that are appropriate for patients who have a loss of mobility or function.

TABLE 4–1: NURSING DIAGNOSES FOR PATIENTS WITH A LOSS OF MOBILITY OR FUNCTION

- Activity intolerance related to decreased muscle strength and tone
- Knowledge deficit about immobility and potential complications
- Altered peripheral tissue perfusion related to immobility and constriction from immobilization devices (traction, casts, splints, braces, etc.)
- Impaired skin integrity related to bedrest or pressure from immobilization devices (traction, casts, splints, braces, etc.)
- Risk for infection related to immobility, possible surgical intervention
- Self-care deficit (feeding, bathing, toileting, etc.) related to loss of mobility and functional ability

Adapted from: Eggenberger, S. (1998). Knowledge base for patients with musculoskeletal dysfunction. In F. Monahan & M. Neighbors (Eds.) *Medical-surgical nursing: Foundations for clinical practice*, 2nd ed., pp. 837-886. Philadelphia: W. B. Saunders Co.

MUSCULOSKELETAL PAIN

The most common symptom of musculoskeletal disorders is pain (Schoen, 2000). The pain may be acute or chronic in nature and is frequently accompanied by other clinical manifestations such as swelling, deformity, inflammation, or muscle spasms (Gordon, 1998). The orthopedic nurse must be competent in assessing and managing pain control and evaluating the patient's response to interventions designed to relieve pain and promote comfort. It is important for the nurse to remember that pain is a subjective experience that can only be described by the person who is experiencing it.

Pain can occur in the joint, muscle, or bone (Eggenberger, 1998). It can be highly variable in quality depending upon the cause and location. Joint pain is frequently due to inflammation or damaged joint structure and is aggravated by movement. Bone pain tends to manifest itself as an aching or throbbing pain. It may be localized or more diffuse. If the bone pain is due to an infection, as in osteomyelitis, the pain is likely to be severe. Muscle pain may manifest itself as an ache and be aggravated by movement, or it may be acute, as in a muscle sprain or spasm.

Because of the wide variations of pain that can occur in musculoskeletal disorders and the subjective nature of the pain experience, it is important that the nurse carefully assess each patient to determine the location, quality, severity, duration, and precipitating factors related to the pain (Schoen, 2000). The nurse should also assess the factors that alleviate or aggravate the patient's pain. The use of a pain assessment scale can help quantify the level of pain that the patient is experiencing. The patient's self-reporting of the pain is considered the most reliable indicator (Eggenberger, 1998).

In addition to assessing the patient's pain, the nurse should also assess for other signs and symptoms that might accompany the pain. These signs

TABLE 4–2: NURSING INTERVENTIONS FOR PATIENTS WITH LOSS OF MOBILITY OR FUNCTION

Activity intolerance	Impaired skin integrity
Schedule frequent rest periods	Inspect skin frequently
Alternate periods of rest with planned activities	Implement measures to decrease skin friction/ pressure from bed and immobilization devices
Active or passive range-of-motion exercises	Alter position frequently
Isometric exercises	Aseptic technique for dressing changes
Arrange environment so frequently used items are nearby	Risk for infection
Develop exercise program (PT, OT)	Monitor vital signs
Explore lifestyle changes	Incentive spirometry; coughing, deep breathing
Knowledge deficit	Increase fluid intake
Altered peripheral tissue perfusion	Monitor intake and output
Alter position frequently	Encourage well-balanced diet high in protein and vitamins
Range-of-motion exercises	
Anti-embolism stockings	Aseptic technique for pin site care and wound care
Pneumatic compression devices	Self-care deficit
Assess for signs of thrombosis	Use adaptive equipment as necessary
Frequent neurovascular checks	Provide assistance with ADL as needed
Assess for circulatory impairment due to immobilization devices	Safe use of ambulatory devices
	Consult with OT and PT
Avoid pressure behind knees	Home health care
Stop smoking	

Teach patient and family about:

- Hazards of immobility
- Increase fluid intake and fiber in diet
- Deep breathing and coughing
- Inspection and care of skin

- Correct application of immobilization devices
- Maintenance of safe home environment
- When to seek medical advice

and symptoms may provide an indication of the etiology of the pain. The nurse should inspect the area for redness or deformity and gently palpate for warmth, tenderness, or swelling. Affected joints should be carefully placed through range-of-motion exercises to determine if there are any limitations. If a fracture or joint dislocation is a possibility, the nurse should not attempt to move the affected body part. Instead, the nurse should question the patient about how the pain interferes with mobility or the performance of activities of daily living (Eggenberger, 1998).

Two groups who require special consideration when assessing pain are children and the elderly (Gordon, 1998). Because children may not readily acknowledge that they are experiencing pain, it is sometimes assumed that they are not in pain. This does a grave injustice to these children. Nurses must assess children for pain in a manner that is appropriate for their developmental level. Visual analog scales with "smiley" faces or "unhappy" faces may be helpful in assessing pain levels. Many young children do not understand the term "pain;" communicating with children using terms they understand is essential.

The elderly are frequently undertreated for pain. They may be reluctant to express pain, fearing that they will be labeled an uncooperative patient or assuming that pain, such as that experienced in arthritis, is a normal part of aging and they simply have to accept its existence. Some may be confused and unable to communicate their needs. In addition, some health care providers still believe that older people have less sensitivity to pain or may not be able to safely tolerate pain medications. It is important that the nurse correct any misconceptions about pain and pain treatment that may be held by the patient or the nurse's colleagues.

Pain may be treated by pharmacological and non-pharmacological methods. Table 4–3 describes nursing interventions that are appropriate for patients who are experiencing pain related to musculoskeletal disorders.

SUMMARY

In order to provide safe, quality nursing care the orthopedic nurse needs an understanding of the common clinical manifestations associated with musculoskeletal disorders. The most common clinical manifestations associated with musculoskeletal disorders are pain, the loss of mobility, and the loss of function. This chapter provided an overview of each of these problems, along with appropriate nursing interventions. Throughout this course, the reader will receive more in-depth information about each of these patient problems. The general overview in this chapter provides the nurse with a foundation of general nursing care that is applicable to all patients, regardless of the clinical problem.

TABLE 4–3: NURSING INTERVENTIONS FOR PATIENTS WHO ARE EXPERIENCING MUSCULOSKELETAL PAIN

- Pain related to pathophysiological alterations in the musculoskeletal system
- Assess pain — location, location, quality, severity, duration, precipitating, aggravating and alleviating factors
- Maintain patient in proper body alignment
- Ensure that immobilization devices are correctly applied (casts, braces, traction, slings, splints)
- Apply heat and cold therapy safely
- Administer pain medications as needed on a regularly scheduled basis
- Teach patient how to effectively use patient-controlled analgesia
- Implement non-pharmacological means of pain control in conjunction with pain medication (mental imagery, massage, distraction, relaxation techniques, music therapy)
- Evaluate patient's response to pain medication and other interventions

CHAPTER 4
Questions 21-23

21. The nurse's initial assessment of any patient with a musculoskeletal disorder should include the patient's

    a. ability to perform self-care activities.
    b. long-term goals for rehabilitation.
    c. history of alcohol intake.
    d. family history of autoimmune disorders.

22. When assessing the pain a patient is experiencing from rheumatoid arthritis, the nurse should remember that

    a. elderly patients feel pain less intensely than younger individuals.
    b. the amount of pain the patient is experiencing can be validated by the loss of function.
    c. the patient's self-reporting of pain is the most reliable indicator available to the nurse.
    d. observing the patient's nonverbal behaviors can help determine the severity of the patient's pain.

23. When caring for a patient who is experiencing activity intolerance due to decreased muscle strength, the most appropriate nursing intervention would be to

    a. assess the patient for neurovascular impairment.
    b. help the patient plan a schedule for activities and rest periods.
    c. encourage the patient to complete all activities early in the morning.
    d. administer oxygen before engaging in any activity.

CHAPTER 5

DIAGNOSTIC TESTS FOR MUSCULOSKELETAL DISORDERS

CHAPTER OBJECTIVE

After completing this chapter, the reader will be able to describe the tests used to diagnose disorders of the musculoskeletal system, as well as the nursing care associated with the procedures.

LEARNING OBJECTIVES

After studying this chapter, the reader will be able to

1. specify the radiologic procedures used to diagnose musculoskeletal disorders.

2. identify the laboratory procedures used to diagnose musculoskeletal disorders.

3. indicate the nursing care associated with diagnostic tests of the musculoskeletal system.

OVERVIEW

Diagnostic tests of the musculoskeletal system provide important objective data that aid in the diagnosis of various musculoskeletal disorders. Diagnostic tests include radiologic procedures and/or laboratory procedures, often consisting of serum, blood, or urine studies. The radiologic procedures may be invasive or non-invasive in nature. The most common radiologic procedure used for diagnosing musculoskeletal disorders is the non-invasive x-ray. Laboratory tests provide information about the patient's complete blood count, blood

chemistry levels, muscle enzyme levels, and urine. The nurse is responsible for knowing the normal values of the laboratory tests and understanding the significance of abnormal findings. It is important that the nurse also understand the nursing care that is associated with the procedures. This chapter describes the tests used to diagnose problems of the musculoskeletal system and the nursing care associated with those tests.

NON-INVASIVE RADIOLOGIC PROCEDURES

Radiography

Radiography is the most common non-invasive diagnostic procedure used for identifying musculoskeletal disorders (Doheny & Sedlak, 2001). Radiography studies, or x-rays, are used to assess the structural integrity of the bones or joints. X-rays can reveal fractures of bones or joint structure changes. X-rays are usually taken from an anteroposterior and/or lateral view, and they can be taken and evaluated relatively quickly. X-rays require no special preparation of the patient, beyond removing any radiopaque articles in the vicinity of the body part being x-rayed (e.g. necklaces, rings) that may cause a visual interference with the results. The nurse should explain the procedure to the patient and the importance of not moving while the x-ray is being taken.

Computed Tomography Scan (CT Scan)

The CT scan provides a detailed 3-dimensional picture of musculoskeletal body structures (Ruda, 2000a). As a result, CT scans are used to diagnose fractures in areas that are difficult to x-ray and can also be used to diagnose soft tissue injuries, trauma to ligaments and tendons, and tumors (Liddel, 2000a). CT scans require no special preparation of the patient beyond informing the patient to lie still during the procedure. A CT scan may take a little longer to complete than the routine x-ray. Sometimes contrast agents may be used to provide better visualization of a body part. In these cases, it is important to assess the patient for any allergies to iodine or seafood prior to the use of the contrast agent.

Magnetic Resonance Imaging (MRI)

MRI uses radio waves and magnetic fields to visualize abnormalities of soft tissue. MRI is particularly helpful in diagnosing ligament, muscle, tendon, and cartilage injuries (Liddel, 2000a). Because of the electromagnetic forces involved in MRI, it is important that *all* metal objects, no matter how small, be removed from the patient prior to the procedure. If the patient has metal implants or clips of any type, he or she will not be an appropriate candidate for MRI. MRI is painless, but for some patients, it can be an anxiety-producing experience. The patient must lie still for approximately 1–2 hours while positioned inside a chamber. For patients who are claustrophobic, this can be extremely difficult. Anti-anxiety medication might be needed to help the patient tolerate the procedure. The nurse should also inform the patient of the noise the equipment makes during the scanning procedure, so that the patient is not startled when the sound begins.

Bone Densitometry

Bone densitometry is used to measure bone density and diagnose the presence of osteoporosis. It can also be used to measure the patient's response to treatment of osteoporosis. Dual-energy x-ray absorptiometry (DEXA) is a common type of bone densitometry that is used to measure bone mass. Measurements of bone mass are taken at the spine, hip, or wrist. DEXA is an accurate and quick form of density measurement. Bone sonometry, which uses ultrasound, is another form of bone densitometry that measures bone density at the heel bone (Liddel, 2000a). The nurse should inform the patient that bone measurement procedures are painless and relatively quick. They require no special patient preparation.

INVASIVE RADIOLOGIC PROCEDURES

Bone Scan

The bone scan is a radioisotope study that is used to detect a variety of musculoskeletal disorders. A radioisotope is injected into the patient intravenously and is taken up in the bone. The isotope will eventually concentrate in areas of bone that have an increased blood flow. Examples of pathological bone conditions that lead to an increased uptake of the isotope include osteomyelitis, pathological fractures, osteoporosis, and bone malignancies. Decreased blood flow to the bone will lead to decreased uptake of the isotope (Doheny & Sedlak, 2001). Avascular necrosis is an example of a musculoskeletal disorder that will show evidence of a decreased isotope uptake.

Nursing care prior to a bone scan includes assessing the patient for allergies to iodine or seafood before administering the isotope and encouraging the patient to drink large amounts of fluid to encourage the circulation and eventual elimination of the isotope. The isotope is administered about 2–3 hours before the scan. The bone scan will take approximately 1 hour, so the nurse should be sure to have the patient void before the procedure. The patient will be asked to lie supine during the scan. The procedure is painless. The nurse should also reassure the patient that the isotope is harmless. Following the scan, the nurse should continue to encourage the patient to drink large amounts of fluid to promote elimination of the isotope.

Arthrogram

The arthrogram is a radiologic study used to evaluate the structure of a joint cavity. It is typically used to diagnose traumatic ligament and joint capsule injuries, most commonly of the shoulder or knee. An arthrogram involves the injection of air or a contrast agent into the joint capsule to provide an outline of the joint cavity and soft tissue structures. A local anesthetic will be used to minimize any discomfort from the injection. It is important that the injection into the joint be made using aseptic technique to prevent introduction of microorganisms into the joint. After injection of the air or contrast media, a series of x-rays are taken of the joint while it is put through the normal range of motion. Moving the joint distributes the contrast media throughout the joint and reveals on the x-ray any structural damage the joint may have experienced. Following the procedure, the patient is instructed to avoid strenuous use of the joint for approximately 48 hours (Doheny & Sedlak, 2001). A mild analgesic may be prescribed to treat any discomfort the patient may experience. The patient should also be instructed to report any feelings of warmth, increasing pain, redness, swelling in the joint, or elevated temperature, as these can be indications of infection.

Arthroscopy

An arthroscopy allows the physician to directly view joint structures. This procedure is commonly used to diagnose and treat injuries to the ligaments, meniscus, and cartilage. An arthroscopy is usually an outpatient procedure. Under sterile conditions in the operating room, a local anesthetic is first injected into the joint. The joint cavity is then inflated with sterile normal saline, and the arthroscope is inserted into the joint through a small puncture wound. After the procedure, the wound is covered with a sterile dressing and the patient may be instructed to restrict activity for a few days postoperatively. Analgesics will be prescribed for postoperative discomfort. Potential complications of an arthroscopy may include infection, thrombophlebitis, joint effusion, neurovascular compromise, and hemarthrosis (Liddel, 2000a). The patient should be instructed to report any signs of swelling or infection.

Arthrocentesis

An arthrocentesis is the aspiration of synovial fluid from a joint, most commonly the knee, for the purpose of diagnosing joint disease or removing fluid from joint to decrease pain. It may also be used to instill medication into a joint. Synovial fluid is normally a clear, light, straw-colored fluid. There are usually only small amounts of synovial fluid present in a joint. However, in certain diseases, such as rheumatoid arthritis or septic arthritis, the synovial fluid becomes cloudy and increases in volume as a result of inflammation and possibly infection in the joint. Bacteria and increased WBCs and protein may also be found in the synovial fluid of an inflamed or infected joint. Nursing care following an arthrocentesis includes instructing the patient to rest the joint for approximately 24 hours. Frequently the joint will be wrapped with an Ace bandage during this time period (Marek, 1999a).

Electromyogram (EMG)

An electromyogram measures the electrical activity of skeletal muscles. It involves inserting small gauge electrode needles into the skeletal muscle and providing a mild electrical stimulus to the muscle. The resulting electrical activity of the muscles is recorded. The electromyogram is used to evaluate muscle weakness or pain and to differentiate between neurological and muscular disorders. The EMG is most commonly used to detect primary muscle disease or lower motor neuron disorders (Ruda, 2000a). Patients may fear having an EMG and worry that they will receive a severe shock from the electrical stimulus. The nurse should reassure the patient that the procedure is safe. However, the procedure can produce some discomfort, and the patient may require a mild analgesic upon completion of the test.

Myelogram

The myelogram is an invasive radiologic study of the spinal subarachnoid space. It is performed to visualize disorders of the spinal canal such as spinal stenosis, tumors, or a herniated nucleus pulposus. In recent times with the advent of MRI and the CT scan, myelograms are performed less frequently (Marek, 1999a). However, they may still have some benefit if other studies are inconclusive or contraindicated. Myelograms are most frequently performed on the lumbar region of the spinal column.

To perform the myelogram, the patient is placed in a sitting or lateral position, a lumbar puncture is performed, and a radiopaque substance is injected into the subarachnoid space. This substance is either oil- or water-based. The oil-based substance is more viscous than the water-based medium. The water-based contrast medium is most commonly used, as there are fewer complications with the water-based medium than the oil-based medium. The most common complication of the oil-based medium is severe headaches following the procedure. The water-based contrast medium is more likely to cause nausea, vomiting, and headaches. Patients may also experience allergic reactions to the medium, so emergency equipment should be available during the procedure.

The myelogram is an outpatient procedure, with the patient usually being admitted to the hospital the morning of the procedure. Nursing care prior to a myelogram includes providing patient education so that the patient knows what to expect during the procedure. The nurse should find out if the patient has any allergies to shellfish or iodine, as this would be a contraindication to receiving the contrast medium. In addition, if the patient is going to receive a water-based contrast medium, he or she should be told not to take any amphetamines, tricyclic antidepressants, or phenothiazides for 12 hours prior to the procedure (Marek, 1999a). These medications may lower the patient's seizure threshold and predispose the patient to experiencing seizures. The patient must be instructed to maintain NPO after a clear liquid breakfast. Sedatives may be administered prior to the procedure to help alleviate anxiety. A local anesthetic will be used prior to the lumbar puncture being performed. Post-procedure nursing care is summarized in Table 5–1.

TABLE 5–1: POST-MYELOGRAM NURSING CARE

- Encourage fluids to aid in elimination of contrast medium, decrease likelihood of headache, and replace cerebrospinal fluid
- If oil medium was used, maintain bed rest for 8 hours in flat, supine position
- If water medium was used, maintain bed rest for 3 hours (or as prescribed) with head elevated 30 degrees
- Assess lumbar puncture site for bleeding
- Observe patient for side effects to contrast medium — nausea, vomiting, headache
- Perform neurological checks and monitor vital signs
- Instruct patient to avoid lifting for 24 hours, report any signs of infection, any drainage from the lumbar puncture, and any photophobia, persistent nausea, or vomiting

(Ahearn-Spera, 2000) (Marek, 1999)

LABORATORY PROCEDURES

The laboratory procedures that may be performed to diagnose musculoskeletal problems include urine tests and blood work that include evaluation of various serologic studies, muscle enzymes, and mineral metabolism.

Common urinary tests to diagnose musculoskeletal disorders include 24-hour urine tests for uric acid or creatine-creatinine ratio. Uric acid may be elevated in the urine of patients who have gouty arthritis. The creatine-creatinine ratio is increased in muscular disease, as the kidneys begin to excrete increased amounts of creatine due to the muscles' decreased ability to convert creatine (Marek, 1999a). Urinary calcium levels will be increased in skeletal disorders that cause release of calcium due to bone destruction (Liddel, 2000a).

Muscle enzymes are released from damaged muscle cells and are therefore elevated in the blood stream. Two enzymes that are released when muscles are damaged are creatine kinase and aspartate aminotransferase (AST). Aldolase is most commonly elevated in muscular dystrophy (Liddel, 2000a).

The mineral metabolism of calcium, phosphorus, and alkaline phosphatase can be altered in a variety of musculoskeletal conditions (Ruda, 2000a). For example, serum calcium levels are elevated in bone cancer, multiple myeloma, and immobility. Serum calcium levels are decreased in osteoporosis and osteomalacia. Serum phosphorus levels have an inverse relationship to calcium levels and are decreased in musculoskeletal disorders that cause increased serum calcium levels. Alkaline phosphatase levels are elevated in disorders that lead to increased osteoblastic activity, such as bone cancer, healing fractures, and osteoporosis.

Other commonly ordered serology studies in musculoskeletal disorders include nonspecific blood tests for substances that may be elevated in inflammation and infection, such as the erythrocyte sedimentation rate (ESR) and C-reactive protein. An elevated antinuclear antibody (ANA) level may indicate the presence of rheumatoid arthritis or systemic lupus erythematosus. Rheumatoid factor (RF) is another nonspecific study; when RF is present in the blood, it may indicate the presence of rheumatoid arthritis and connective tissue disease (Ruda, 2000a). Complete blood counts may be performed to detect any decrease in the patient's hemoglobin and hematocrit levels resulting from blood loss or

any elevation in white blood count to indicate infection. Table 5–2 lists the normal values of common serum blood studies used to diagnose musculoskeletal disorders.

TABLE 5–2: NORMAL LABORATORY VALUES OF BLOOD TESTS FOR MUSCULOSKELETAL DISORDERS

Laboratory Test	Normal Values
Serum calcium	9–11 mg/dl
Serum phosphorus	2.8–4.5 mg/dl
Alkaline phosphatase	20–90 U/L
Creatine kinase	Men: 5–55 U/L; Women 5–35 U/L
Aldolase	1.0–7.5 U/L
Aspartate aminotransferase	15–45 U/L
Erythrocyte sedimentation rate (ESR)	<20 mm/hr
Antinuclear antibody (ANA)	Negative
C-reactive protein (CRP)	Negative
Rheumatoid factor (RF)	Negative

SUMMARY

There are a variety of non-invasive and invasive radiologic procedures and laboratory tests that may be used to diagnose the presence of musculoskeletal disorders or disease. These tests provide objective data that will be useful in determining the patient's treatment and plan of care. As the majority of these procedures are performed on an outpatient basis, it is important that the patient receives the information necessary to ensure that he or she can safely perform self-care activities in the home setting. The nurse assumes primary responsibility for patient education before and after the diagnostic procedures.

EXAM QUESTIONS

CHAPTER 5
Questions 24-28

24. A patient scheduled to undergo a magnetic resonance imaging (MRI) test should be instructed to

    a. be NPO for 8 hours prior to the test.

    b. remove all metal objects prior to the test.

    c. lie flat for 3 hours following the test.

    d. keep the puncture site dry following the test.

25. The test that is used to effectively measure a patient's bone density is the

    a. bone scan.

    b. skeletal x-ray.

    c. CT scan.

    d. DEXA.

26. The primary purpose of the arthroscopy is to

    a. allow direct visualization of joint structures.

    b. aspirate synovial fluid from a joint.

    c. inject corticosteroids directly into a joint.

    d. observe joint movement.

27. A common urinary test used to diagnose musculoskeletal disorders is

    a. urine culture and sensitivity.

    b. urinalysis.

    c. 24-hour urine collection for uric acid

    d. urine specific gravity.

28. A patient who has just returned from a myelogram procedure that was performed with a water-based contrast medium should be

    a. restricted in fluid intake for 3 hours following the procedure.

    b. placed on seizure precautions.

    c. placed in bed with the head elevated at 30 degrees.

    d. given anti-anxiety medication.

CHAPTER 6

TREATMENT INTERVENTIONS FOR PATIENTS WITH MUSCULOSKELETAL DISORDERS

CHAPTER OBJECTIVE

After completing this chapter, the reader will be able to describe the various treatment interventions that are used when caring for patients who have experienced musculoskeletal trauma.

LEARNING OBJECTIVES

After studying this chapter, the reader will be able to

1. indicate how to safely apply heat and cold therapy.

2. differentiate the various types of casts.

3. select the proper nursing care of a patient who has a cast.

4. specify the principles of traction therapy.

5. indicate the different types of traction.

6. choose the proper nursing care of the patient who has traction.

7. indicate the various complications associated with traction and casts.

8. specify the proper nursing care of a patient who has an external fixation device.

OVERVIEW

Patients who have experienced musculoskeletal trauma frequently require immobilization of the injured body part to prevent further injury and to promote healing. Common methods of immobilization include the application of a cast or the use of traction. In some instances, the injury may require the use of an external fixation device to achieve adequate immobilization of the injured area. Heat and cold therapy may also be used to help relieve pain and promote healing. The orthopedic nurse is responsible for understanding the principles of care related to each of these interventions and providing safe nursing care. This chapter addresses the treatment interventions used when caring for a patient with musculoskeletal trauma and the nursing responsibilities associated with each intervention.

APPLICATION OF HEAT AND COLD THERAPY

Heat and cold therapy are frequently used in the treatment of a variety of musculoskeletal disorders, especially when the patient has experienced trauma. The nurse is responsible for safely administering heat and cold therapy. When incorrectly applied, either therapy can lead to further tissue damage and impair healing.

Heat therapy is used to promote healing, decrease pain, and support the inflammatory process. The local application of heat causes vasodilation in the area where the heat is applied. The vasodilation effect leads to an increase in tissue metabolism and an increase in capillary permeability. As a result, there is increased blood flow to the area that brings nutrients to the injured tissues and removes waste materials. Because of the increased blood flow, venous congestion in the injured area is decreased, which helps decrease edema. The warmth of the heat therapy also relaxes muscles and decreases the pain that may occur due to muscle spasms (Ayello & Perry, 2001). Examples of musculoskeletal conditions that can be treated with the application of heat therapy can be found in Table 6–1.

TABLE 6–1: EXAMPLES OF MUSCULOSKELETAL CONDITIONS TREATED BY HEAT THERAPY
Muscle strain
Low back pain
Arthritis
Osteomyelitis
Joint pain
Edematous area

Cold therapy is used to decrease pain and minimize the development of edema. The local application of cold causes vasoconstriction in the areas where the cold is applied. As a result, the blood flow to the area is reduced, thus decreasing the development of edema. The cold also produces a local anesthetic effect, which decreases the sensation of pain (Ayello & Perry, 2001). Examples of musculoskeletal conditions that can be treated with the application of cold therapy can be found in Table 6–2.

TABLE 6–2: EXAMPLES OF MUSCULOSKELETAL CONDITIONS TREATED BY COLD THERAPY
Arthritis
Fractures
Sprains and strains*
Muscle spasms
Joint injury*

* (at time of injury)

Either heat or cold therapy can result in further damage to tissue if not properly applied. Heat therapy should not be applied to any area that is actively bleeding, as the heat and vasodilation effect will promote continued bleeding. The heat must be carefully regulated to avoid burning or blistering the skin. The patient should be cautioned not to increase the temperature setting. Prolonged application of heat should also be avoided because after about 1 hour of application, a reflex vasoconstriction will develop. The reflex vasoconstriction is a protective response by the body to try to conserve body heat that is being lost through vasodilation. Periodically removing the heat source will prevent the occurrence of the reflex vasoconstriction and will also allow the nurse to closely inspect the skin for any tissue damage. The nurse should observe the skin for any signs of tenderness, any redness that does not quickly recede after removal of the heat, or any signs of blistering (Ayello & Perry, 2001).

Cold therapy should not be applied to any area that has already developed edema. The vasoconstriction that occurs as a result of the cold decreases circulation and will hinder the removal of excess fluid from the tissues. Cold therapy can also cause tissues to freeze if the skin is not carefully protected from the cold source. Prolonged application of cold should be avoided as it can lead to reflex vasodilation. This is a protective response by the body to avoid the tissue ischemia that can develop over time as a result of the vasoconstriction and decreased blood flow produced by the cold therapy. The nurse should periodically remove the cold application and carefully inspect the skin for tissue damage. Skin that is developing damage from the cold application will initially look red and then become mottled in appearance. The patient may complain of burning pain and numbness in the area (Ayello & Perry, 2001).

Safety precautions that should be implemented when applying either cold or heat therapy include first carefully inspecting the skin in the affected area and noting any alterations in skin integrity. The nurse will want to carefully assess the condition of the skin following the treatment as well. All equipment should be carefully inspected to ensure safe functioning. The nurse should instruct the patient to not adjust any temperature settings and to report immediately any feelings of discomfort. If the patient cannot accurately detect temperature changes in the skin due to previously existing medical conditions or altered mental status, the nurse will need to frequently assess the skin during the course of the application. All treatments should be carefully timed, adhering to the prescribed length of time for the therapy. The nurse documents the therapy, including the length of time it was applied, the appearance of the area following the therapy, and the patient's response.

As many patients who receive heat and cold therapy are treated as outpatients, it is important that the nurse teach the safe administration of heat and cold to patients and their significant others. Patients should be taught how to safely apply the therapy, the time limits for each application, and how to assess the skin before, during and after each application.

CARE OF THE PATIENT WITH A CAST

Casts, which are a type of external fixation device, are used to immobilize a specific area of the body that has been injured. Most frequently used to immobilize fractures, casts may also be used to treat soft tissue injuries. The application of a cast stabilizes the injured area and prevents movement so that healing can occur, while typically allowing the patient to retain mobility (Liddel, 2000b).

Casts are made of various materials and thickness. The choice of cast will depend upon the condition being treated. The cast will usually extend from the joint proximal to the injury to the joint distal to the injury, so that complete immobilization of the injured area can be accomplished (Liddel,

2000b). The most common types of casts are illustrated in Figure 6–1.

Short arm casts are used to immobilize wrist or metacarpal fractures. Long arm casts are used to immobilize elbow and forearm fractures. Short leg casts are applied to ankle and foot injuries, while long leg casts are used to immobilize a fractured tibia or knee injury. Long leg casts may also be used for unstable ankle fractures. Body jacket casts are used to stabilize thoracic or lumbar spinal injuries. The hip spica cast is used to immobilize femoral fractures and is frequently used in children. The spica cast may be single or double depending upon the location and extent of the fracture (Ruda, 2000b).

Casts can also be used as splints where they are used to immobilize a body part without completely encasing it. Cast braces, which permit joint mobility, can also be used. With a cast brace, two casts are made — one for application above a joint and one for application below a joint. The two casts are joined together by hinges that permit mobility of the joint (Marek, 1999b).

Application of the Cast

Following the reduction of the fracture, a cast will be applied. The type of material used to make the cast may be of plaster or various synthetic materials such as fiberglass or plastic. Plaster is the traditional casting material and is relatively inexpensive. It is also heavier and takes longer to dry after application. Plaster must be kept dry after application. The fiberglass or synthetic materials are lighter in weight, quick to dry, and can tolerate submersion in water without loss of form or strength. The type of cast material selected will depend upon the type of injury. Synthetic casts are more suitable for simple, non-displaced fractures that have little swelling. They also hold up well for long-term use (Dingley, 1999).

The casting materials are available in individual rolls. The rolls are individually submerged in water until they are wet and then unrolled and wrapped around the injured body part. The wrapping process

FIGURE 6-1: COMMON CASTS USED TO TREAT MUSCULOSKELETAL DISORDERS

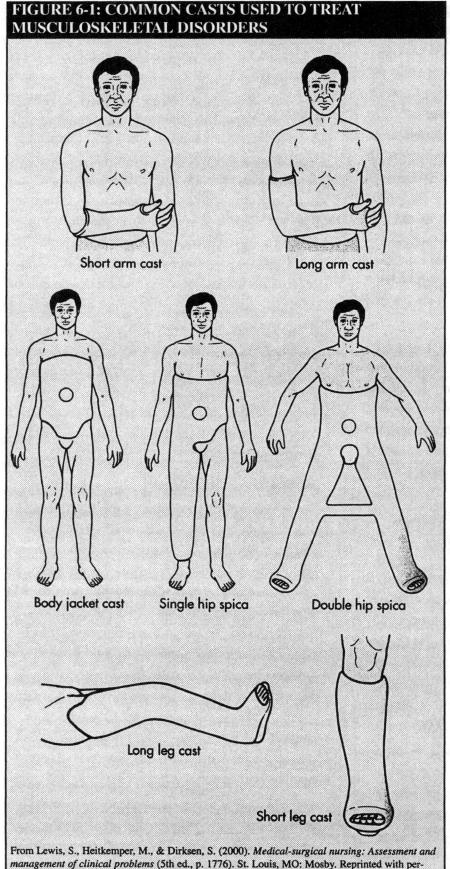

Short arm cast

Long arm cast

Body jacket cast

Single hip spica

Double hip spica

Long leg cast

Short leg cast

From Lewis, S., Heitkemper, M., & Dirksen, S. (2000). *Medical-surgical nursing: Assessment and management of clinical problems* (5th ed., p. 1776). St. Louis, MO: Mosby. Reprinted with permission from Elsevier.

is similar to applying an Ace wrap or other circular bandage. The number of wraps or layers of material will determine the ultimate strength of the cast (Ruda, 2000b). As the material begins to dry, heat is generated and felt by the patient.

Prior to the application of a cast, the nurse may be responsible for preparing the patient's skin. The nurse should clean the skin thoroughly and note any breaks in skin integrity. Disinfectant may be applied to any lesions. The nurse then applies cotton padding material to prevent direct contact of the casting material with the skin. Extra padding may also be placed over any bony prominences to decrease pressure from the cast and help prevent the development of pressure ulcers. A stockinette material is then placed over the padding to hold it in place and to provide the skin with protection from the cast edges. It is important that these materials be applied without wrinkles to prevent areas of pressure and skin breakdown (Roberts, 2001).

After the application of the cast, special precautions should be taken until the cast has dried completely. Drying time will vary dependent upon the type of casting material used. Plaster of Paris takes the longest to dry, requiring 24–48 hours to completely dry and permit weight-bearing (Ruda, 2000b). Plaster will harden in approximately 15 minutes, but it takes much longer for the multiple layers to completely dry. Synthetic casts require about 30 minutes to dry completely (Roberts,

2001). During the cast drying time, regardless of the material used, the patient should be told to expect the sensation of heat.

The nurse should instruct the patient to leave the cast open to air while drying, as keeping it covered will slow the drying process. Covering the cast will also lead to a build-up of heat, which may burn the patient. A wet cast should be manipulated as little as possible to prevent misshaping it. The wet cast should be rested on a pillow that will provide a soft surface and should only be handled by the palms of your hands while being moved. Avoid picking the cast up by your fingertips to decrease the potential for applying pressure, forming indentures, and mis-shaping the cast. Mishandling the cast can lead to the development of pressure areas on the underlying skin. Turning the patient every 2 hours so that a new portion of the cast can be exposed to air will help facilitate consistent drying of all areas of the cast (Ruda, 2000b). Do not use a blow dryer to help dry the cast, as the heat can cause the cast to crack and the patient may also experience a burn (Roberts, 2001). However, a fan can be used to circulate air over the cast.

General Nursing Care Following Cast Application

Nursing care following a cast application includes assessing for complications. The most common complication after the application of a cast is neurovascular compromise due to edema and constriction by the cast. Compartment syndrome can develop. The extremity should be kept elevated above heart level for the first 24–48 hours to decrease the development of edema. An arm that is casted should be rested in a sling with the fingers elevated above the elbow. The nurse should careful-ly perform neurovascular checks on the affected extremity every 30 minutes for the first 4 hours fol-lowing the application of the cast (Dingley, 1999). Routine neurovascular checks are then performed every 4 hours. Neurovascular checks include check-ing pulse, sensation, movement, color, and temper-

ature of the affected extremity distal to the cast. Comparing assessment findings for the affected extremity to the unaffected extremity will help the nurse determine if assessment findings are within normal limits for the patient.

Another aspect of the neurovascular check is assessing for the presence of pain. Pain upon pas-sive movement indicates the presence of neurovas-cular compromise; it must be promptly reported and intervention taken to relieve the compromise. Increasing pain following the application of a cast can be indicative of swelling and constriction from the cast. If the nurse suspects that the patient is developing neurovascular compromise or compart-ment syndrome, treatment cannot be delayed. Delaying treatment means risking permanent irre-versible muscle and nerve damage. One example of potential nerve damage that can occur in patients with leg casts is injury to the peroneal nerve that lies laterally on the outer aspect of the calf. Damage to the peroneal nerve results in foot drop and will cause the patient to be unable to lift the foot when ambulating. Proper assessment of peripheral nerve function is reviewed in Chapter 3, Table 3–4.

To relieve constriction caused by a cast that has become too tight, the cast should be bivalved, or cut in half along both sides of the cast. Bivalving a cast involves cutting through the cast and the padding underneath. The cast is then spread apart to relieve constriction. After the constriction has been relieved, an Ace bandage can be applied to the cast parts to hold the cast intact and maintain alignment of the fracture. Patients who are being discharged home immediately following the application of a cast should be instructed on how to perform neu-rovascular checks and what indicators require immediate medical attention.

Additional nursing care includes assessing the cast for any drainage, wet spots, or unusual odors. The nurse should circle, date and time any drainage areas observed on the cast and note if the drainage area continues to grow. Sniffing at the edges of the cast can help detect any unusual odors that might indicate the presence of an infection. The nurse should also feel the cast for any areas of heat, as this too, can indicate an infection has developed beneath the cast. The patient who is being discharged soon after the cast has been applied should be instructed to report any of these findings promptly to a health care provider.

Skin care is another important aspect of nursing care after the application of a cast. The skin at the edges of the cast should be routinely inspected for signs of redness and irritation. The cast edges can be covered in adhesive tape or the stockinette can be pulled back over the edges to prevent skin irritation. The skin can be cleansed gently with warm water to remove any cast fragments.

For patients with a lower extremity cast, ambulation and weight-bearing will begin as the physician prescribes. It will be important for the patient to maintain muscle strength by performing isometric exercises such as quadriceps setting and gluteal setting. All unaffected joints should be put through normal range-of-motion exercises. The patient should be encouraged to exercise the toes. Maintaining upper body strength is also important as the patient will need to be able to use assistive devices such as walkers or crutches. When weight-bearing is allowed, a cast boot or walking heel will be used to provide protection to the cast (Marek, 1999b).

For patients with an arm cast, the nurse should encourage the patient to do finger exercises and shoulder exercises as allowed. The patient may experience frustration as he or she tries to accommodate to using one arm to perform activities of daily living. The patient should use a sling whenever ambulating to keep the arm elevated and provide support. It is important that the sling strap be adjusted correctly to avoid placing too much pressure on the cervical spinal nerves. The patient should be told to keep the arm elevated when resting to prevent edema.

Care of the Patient in a Body or Spica Cast

Patients who are in a body cast or spica cast have special needs. Body casts are used to immobilize the spine; hip spica casts are used following some hip surgeries and for treatment of some femoral fractures. Shoulder spica casts are used to treat some humeral neck fractures (Liddel, 2000b). These patients are significantly immobilized and need assistance to meet their daily hygiene needs. They also must be monitored closely for complications that can develop due to immobility. Being encased in a body or spica cast can cause anxiety in some patients. The nurse should explain the procedure to the patient and reassure the patient that his or her needs will be met. Pain medication or medication to reduce anxiety can be administered prior to the procedure.

After application of the cast, the patient will need to be turned every 2 hours to promote drying and ensure that pressure is not placed on any one side of the cast for prolonged periods. It is important that the cast not become misshapened. When turning the patient with a wet cast, it is essential to have enough personnel assist with turning so as to not to damage the cast or twist the patient's body inside the cast. At least three people should assist when turning the patient. If an abductor bar is in place to stabilize the hip spica cast, personnel must know not to turn the patient using the bar (Liddel, 2000b). Ample pillows should be used to position and support the patient and prevent areas of pressure from developing.

The skin of the patient should be assessed daily on each shift to detect any signs of irritation or pressure. Using a flashlight, the nurse can inspect the skin under the edges of the cast and gently clean the skin. The patient should be turned prone several times a day, if not contraindicated, to relieve pressure on the back and promote respiratory functioning. While lying prone, the nurse can place a small pillow under the patient's abdomen to provide support and position the patient's feet so that they hang freely over the edge of the mattress to prevent pressure on the toes. If the patient's feet cannot hang over the edge of the mattress, a pillow can be placed under the feet to lift them from the bed. Patients may have difficulty tolerating the prone position, so they should be monitored closely and the position changed as necessary (Liddel, 2000b).

The perineal area of the cast will have an opening that will allow for daily hygiene care to be administered. The patient will very likely prefer using a fracture bedpan for elimination. The nurse can protect the edges of the cast's perineal opening with a protective plastic sheet to prevent soiling during elimination. Elevating the head of the bed, if allowed, or placing the patient in reverse Trendelenburg position while using the bedpan may assist with elimination. A "window" may also be cut in the cast over the abdominal area to relieve abdominal distention and to allow the nurse access to check for bladder distention (Marek, 1999b). It is important that the patient maintain an adequate fluid intake. Stool softeners may also be prescribed.

Patients who are encased in large casts, such as a body or spica cast, may develop cast syndrome. The patient may feel claustrophobic and anxious, exhibiting signs of autonomic responses. These signs include dilated pupils and increased heart rate, blood pressure, and respirations. Such patients may become diaphoretic. In addition to these responses, the patient may also experience physiologic gastrointestinal problems. These problems develop when the cast compresses the superior mesenteric artery at the duodenum (Ruda, 2000b) or as a result of lying in a supine position for a prolonged period of time (Roberts, 2001). These patients complain of nausea, distention, vomiting, and abdominal pain. Treatment of cast syndrome includes relieving the abdominal pressure by bivalving the cast or cutting a window in the cast over the abdomen. Nasogastric suction may be used to decompress the abdomen, and intravenous fluids should be given until peristalsis returns (Roberts, 2001).

Removal of a Cast

The cast will be removed with the use of a cast cutter. When it is time for the cast to be removed, the nurse should explain the procedure to the patient. Some patients are anxious about the use of the cast cutter and must be reassured that the cutter will not penetrate the skin. The padding underneath the cast is cut with scissors and carefully removed.

The nurse also must prepare the patient for the appearance of the body part after the cast is removed. The skin on the body part will appear dry and scaly; it may itch. The patient should be cautioned not to scratch the skin, as it will be easily irritated. The skin should be gently washed and lotion applied. The body part will also be stiff and weak due to lack of use. The patient should gradually resume normal activity. Physical therapy may be prescribed to assist the patient to regain strength and mobility.

Patient Education for Patients with a Cast

Since many patients who have a cast applied are treated as outpatients and discharged home shortly thereafter, patient education is very important. Emphasizing patient education prior to discharge can help prevent the development of complications.

Table 6–3 describes the education appropriate for a patient with a cast.

CARE OF THE PATIENT IN TRACTION

Traction is used to provide pull to a body part, while countertraction is applied to pull in the opposite direction. Traction is prescribed to treat various musculoskeletal problems. For example, it is used to reduce a fracture and maintain normal alignment of the bone ends. In the treatment of fractures, traction may be applied pre- or post-operatively. Traction is also used to help decrease muscle spasms and contractions, thus decreasing pain. Traction can be used to treat or prevent deformities.

TABLE 6–3: PATIENT EDUCATION FOR A PATIENT WITH A CAST

- Keep affected body part elevated to decrease swelling
- Use analgesics as prescribed to control pain
- Promptly report pain with passive movement or pain that is unrelieved by analgesics and elevation of the body part
- Promptly report any changes in the pulse, sensation, movement, temperature, or color of the affected body part
- Note any cast odors, warm/hot spots on the cast, drainage, or stained cast areas and report promptly
- Report any elevated temperature or feelings of malaise
- Inspect skin at cast edges regularly and report any signs of irritation
- Do not insert anything down inside the cast
- Do not get plaster of Paris casts wet
- Synthetic casts must be dried thoroughly after coming in contact with water
- Do exercises to maintain muscle strength

There are three types of traction — skin, skeletal, and manual. In skin traction, the pull of the weights is applied in an indirect way, directly to the skin. In skeletal traction, a metal pin is inserted into the bone and the weights are then applied directly to the metal pin. Manual traction is applied by the hands and is used to maintain reduction of a fracture while a cast is being applied or other forms of traction are being applied or adjusted.

Traction can also be classified as either running (straight) or balanced suspension traction. For running traction, the affected body part is allowed to rest on the bed with the traction applied in a straight line. With running traction, the patient must maintain his or her position in order to maintain the pull of the traction. Balanced suspension traction, on the other hand, allows the patient to change position in bed while still accurately maintaining the traction

pull. This is achieved by suspending and supporting the affected extremity above the bed with a series of weights and pulleys that maintain the line of pull whenever the patient shifts position (Liddel, 2000c).

Principles of Traction

Traction consists of the application of weights to achieve the desired pull on the affected body part. The physician will prescribe the amount of weight to be applied. The patient's weight and position in bed, and sometimes additional weights, will provide countertraction. Countertraction keeps the patient from being pulled out of bed by the weight of the prescribed traction. The weights are balanced by a system of ropes and pulleys. There are certain principles related to traction that the nurse should implement. These principles can be found in Table 6–4.

TABLE 6–4: PRINCIPLES OF TRACTION

- Patient must be placed in correct body alignment in center of bed to maintain line of pull
- Traction is maintained continuously, unless the physician prescribes otherwise
- Countertraction is maintained continuously
- All ropes must move freely on the pulley at all times
- Rope knots should never touch the pulley
- Ropes should be kept clear of bed linens and any other objects
- Weights must hang freely at all times
- Skeletal traction must never be released

Skin Traction

Skin traction is applied directly to the patient's skin through the use of a traction boot, a traction strip, halters, or belts. Skin traction may be either running traction or balanced suspension traction. Examples of skin traction include Buck's extension traction, Russell's traction, pelvic, and cervical traction. See Figure 6–2 for illustrations of Buck's traction and Figure 6–3 Russell's traction. The amount of weight used in skin traction tends to average 5 to 7 pounds (Roberts, 2001). This amount can usually

FIGURE 6-2: BUCK'S EXTENSION

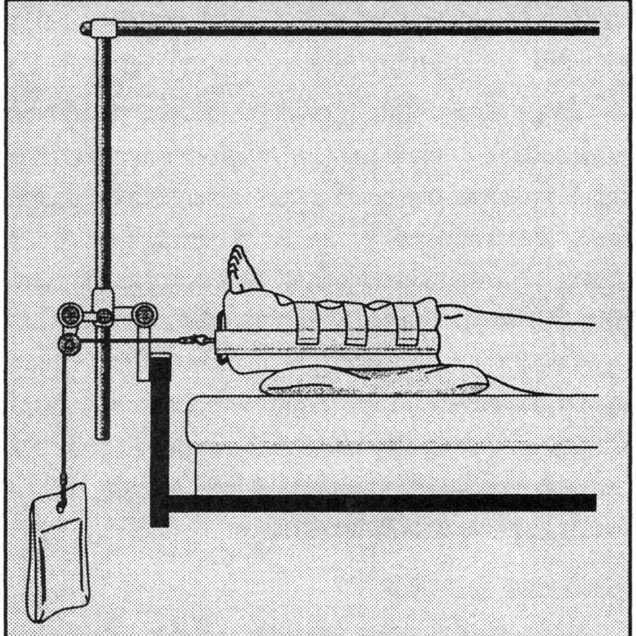

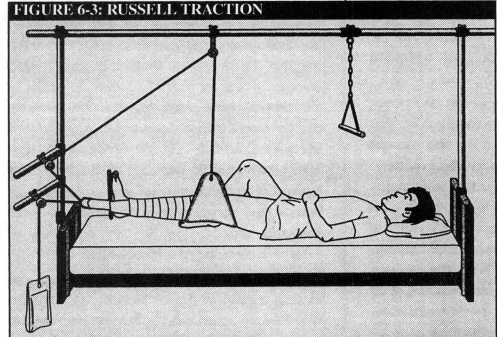

Heel is supported off bed to prevent pressure on heel; weight hangs free of the bed, and foot is well away from footboard of bed. The limb should lie parallel to the bed unless prevented, as in this case, by a slight knee flexion contracture.

From Phipps, W., Sands, J., & Marek, J. (1999). *Medical Surgical Nursing: Concepts and Clinical Practice* (6th ed., p. 1920). St. Louis, MO: Mosby. Reprinted with permission from Elsevier.

FIGURE 6-3: RUSSELL TRACTION

Hip is slightly flexed. Pillows may be used under lower leg to provide support and keep the heel free of the bed.

From Phipps, W., Sands, J., & Marek, J. (1999). *Medical Surgical Nursing: Concepts and Clinical Practice* (6th ed., p. 1920). St. Louis, MO: Mosby. Reprinted with permission from Elsevier.

be applied without placing undue pressure on the patient's skin. Pelvic traction may require more weight (10 to 20 pounds) based upon the patient's weight (Liddel, 2000c). The amount of weight used is also dependent upon the muscle mass of the patient; more weight is needed to overcome muscle spasms in the larger, stronger muscles.

Skin traction is a temporary traction. Continued use of skin traction for a prolonged period of time may result in skin breakdown, most likely over bony prominence areas. Skin breakdown is especially a concern in elderly patients. In some cases, skin traction will be used to temporarily immobilize an injured extremity and minimize muscle spasms prior to surgical treatment, as in a hip fracture (Roberts, 2001). Skin traction is also used to treat muscle spasms that are not associated with fractures, as in lower back pain (pelvic traction) or neck pain (cervical traction). Skin traction may be prescribed continuously or it may be prescribed intermittently. Pelvic and cervical traction are examples of skin traction that are usually prescribed for intermittent intervals.

Buck's extension traction is an example of both skin traction and running traction. This traction is used to immobilize the lower extremities, usually due to a hip fracture. Buck's traction is applied preoperatively to reduce the fracture, maintain alignment, and decrease patient discomfort. Buck's traction may also be used to reduce muscle spasms, treat low back pain, and help correct contractures of the hip and knee (Byrne, 1999). The traction is held in place by traction boots or by straps that are applied to the leg and then secured by an

Ace wrap. The amount of weight applied for Buck's traction is usually 3–8 pounds. The patient's weight and positioning in bed provides countertraction.

Russell's traction is another example of skin traction; it is also an example of balanced suspension traction. Russell's traction allows for the knee to be flexed and suspended in a sling. The traction pull extends horizontally along the leg. This type of traction is most often used to immobilize a fractured tibia (Liddel, 2000b).

There are some contraindications to the application of skin traction. Impaired circulation, skin irritations, wounds, or pressure sores are all potential contraindications. When the nurse applies skin traction, care should be taken to not secure the traction too tightly to the extremity, as this can impair circulation, cause nerve damage, and create pressure sores, especially over the bony prominences. An elderly patient's skin is particularly fragile and prone to breakdown. With traction that is applied to the lower extremities, the nurse should assess carefully for the complication of deep vein thrombosis. Clinical indications of a deep vein thrombosis include redness, warmth, and foot or leg edema. Additionally, the patient may experience calf tenderness or pain in the posterior thigh or popliteal area (Kotch, 2001).

Frequent assessment of the patient is important following the application of skin traction. The nurse should check the traction and do neurovascular checks at least every 2 hours on the affected extremity's fingers or toes (Liddel, 2000b). With patient movement and the pull caused by the traction, it is possible for the traction wrappings to loosen and become ineffective or to tighten and impair circulation and nerve function. The nurse checks pulse, color, temperature, movement, and sensation of the affected body part. The nurse should maintain the patient in good alignment and reposition as necessary. The patient usually lies supine. Preoperatively, the patient with a hip fracture and Buck's traction can be periodically positioned to the affected side

with a pillow between the legs. Turning the patient to the affected side prior to surgical treatment helps to avoid displacement of the fracture fragments.

Once every shift, the skin traction should be removed, and, while manual traction is applied by a second person, the nurse should inspect the skin and bony prominences for areas of redness or break down, cleanse it gently, and then reapply the traction. It is important to be sure that the traction bandages are applied smoothly with no wrinkles that can lead to the development of pressure areas. The nurse should also carefully inspect the patient's back for pressure areas and provide skin care at least every 2 hours to prevent skin break down.

Skeletal Traction

In skeletal traction, the pulling force of the traction is applied directly to a metal pin or wire that has been inserted through the bone. A Steinmann pin or Kirschner wire are the most common examples of pins and wires used for skeletal traction. The use of skeletal traction allows for a direct pull on the bone fragments to achieve alignment. Skeletal traction requires that the patient undergo a surgical procedure to insert the pin or wire into the bone (usually into the distal femur or proximal tibia) so that the traction weights can be applied. Skeletal traction is most commonly used for femoral fractures. Fractures of the cervical spine, humerus, and tibia can also require skeletal traction. More weight is applied with skeletal traction than with skin traction, usually anywhere from 15 to 25 pounds (Liddel, 2000c). This amount of weight is required to overcome muscle spasms and maintain bone alignment. In some instances, additional weight may be needed to achieve the necessary therapeutic effect.

Balanced suspension traction is often used with skeletal traction to support the affected extremity. The Thomas Splint with the Pearson attachment is a form of balanced suspension traction used with lower extremity fractures. Figure 6–4 illustrates this form of traction. The use of balanced suspension

FIGURE 6-4: BALANCED SUSPENSION WITH THOMAS SPLINT AND PEARSON ATTACHMENT.

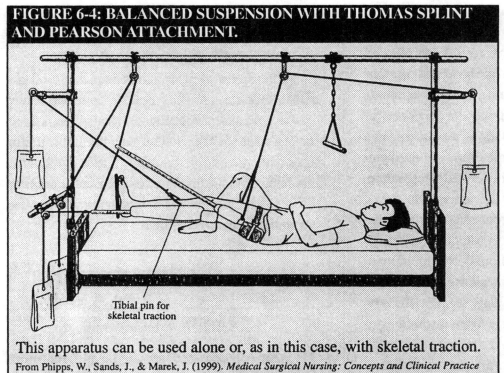

Tibial pin for skeletal traction

This apparatus can be used alone or, as in this case, with skeletal traction.

From Phipps, W., Sands, J., & Marek, J. (1999). *Medical Surgical Nursing: Concepts and Clinical Practice* (6th ed., p. 1921). St. Louis, MO: Mosby. Reprinted with permission from Elsevier.

traction allows the patient more mobility in bed without disrupting the line of traction.

Skeletal traction is never interrupted, as to do so would interfere with the reduction and alignment of the bone fragments. The traction will be removed when callus formation occurs at the fracture site, and it will be replaced with a splint or cast to provide continued support to the affected part (Liddel, 2000c). X-rays are taken periodically to check the progress of bone healing and union at the fracture site. One potential complication of skeletal traction is nonunion of the bone fragments due to too much traction being applied to the extremity, thus keeping the bone fragments separated and preventing union. Too little traction may allow the bone ends to override each other. In addition to showing evidence of healing, X-rays will also reveal the alignment of the bone ends and the effectiveness of the traction.

Another complication associated with skeletal traction is skin breakdown. This breakdown can occur as a result of the patient's position in the bed or as a result of the traction apparatus applying pressure at various points on the affected extremity. The heel of the unaffected extremity, the elbows, and the coccyx are particularly prone to skin breakdown as the patient attempts to shift position in the bed. The nurse should instruct the patient to use an overhead trapeze to facilitate movement and prevent friction on these potential pressure areas. Other areas susceptible to pressure from traction are the bony prominence areas on the affected extremity and any other areas where the traction apparatus rubs against the skin. In the lower extremities, such areas include the heel, popliteal area, Achilles tendon, and ischial tuberosity (Liddel, 2000b). The nurse inspects the skin frequently and adjusts the traction apparatus as needed to avoid pressure areas. The skin should be kept clean and dry.

The neurovascular status of the affected extremity can also be impaired as a result of pressure from the skeletal traction apparatus. Deep vein thrombosis is a potential complication for all immobilized patients, and the balanced suspension traction used with skeletal traction places pressure behind the popliteal area of the leg, further predisposing the patient to decreased circulation and thrombus formation. Pressure can also be placed on the peroneal nerve, leading to foot drop as a result of nerve damage. It is important that the nurse assess the neurovascular status of the affected extremity every 3–4 hours so that staff can promptly intervene if there are any noted pressure areas developing. The nurse also encourages the patient to do active muscle setting exercises to help maintain blood flow in the lower extremities.

Skeletal traction also requires that the nurse provide pin site care to the insertion site of the Steinmann pin or Kirschner wire. These pins or wires are inserted directly into the bone and must be carefully cared for to prevent the introduction of infection into the bone and the development of osteomyelitis. The nurse should assess the pin site each shift for signs of infection — purulent drainage, redness, or pain. An elevated temperature may also be an indication of the onset of an infection at the pin site. A little serous drainage from the pin site is to be anticipated, but other drainage should be promptly reported, and crusting around the insertion site should not be allowed to develop. The nurse cleans the pin site daily as prescribed by the physician; protocols vary from institution to institution. The pin itself should not be manipulated. The pin should not have any movement at the insertion site. If the nurse detects any movement or sliding of the pin, he or she should report this promptly to the physician.

In addition to complications related to the application of traction, patients who have traction applied are also prone to the complications of immobility. Gastrointestinal, urinary, and respiratory complications can develop if the nurse does not monitor the patient closely and implement nursing interventions to prevent the development of complications. Gastrointestinal complications include constipation as a result of the lack of activity, decreased peristalsis, and difficulty using a bedpan. Ensuring an adequate fluid intake and a diet high in fiber can help prevent constipation, as can the use of stool softeners. Urinary tract infections can develop as a result of incomplete emptying of the bladder and difficulty using a bedpan. Increased fluid intake and encouragement to heed the urge to void can help prevent the development of a urinary tract infection. The nurse can facilitate elimination by helping the patient assume as comfortable a position as possible when using the bedpan. To prevent the development of respiratory complications due to immobility, the nurse

should encourage the patient to cough and take deep breaths at regular intervals, as well as using incentive spirometry hourly to fully expand the lungs.

With careful monitoring of the patient's condition, the nurse can prevent the development of many of the potential complications related to skin or skeletal traction. The goal of nursing care is to promote patient comfort, maintain function within the limitations of the traction, and prevent complications so that the patient can regain normal activities when the fracture has healed.

CARE OF THE PATIENT WITH AN EXTERNAL FIXATION DEVICE

External fixation devices are metal frame structures that are externally applied to support and stabilize a fracture. They are used when the patient has suffered an open, complicated fracture with soft tissue injury, and traction or a cast is contraindicated. The external device allows the wound to be treated while the fracture is reduced and held in alignment. It also promotes earlier mobility.

The external fixation device is attached to the bone through the use of a series of pins that are screwed into the bone. Figure 6–5 shows various examples of external fixation devices. External fixation is suitable for use in complicated fractures that occur in the femur, tibia, humerus, forearm, or pelvis (Liddel, 2000).

When the patient has a fracture that requires the application of an external fixation device, the nurse first must prepare the patient for the appearance of the device. The device can be bulky and frightening in appearance with all of the pin insertion sites, and the patient often anticipates that it will be very painful. The patient needs to understand that discomfort related to the use of an external fixator device is minimal; the device actually promotes patient comfort through the stabilization of the frac-

FIGURE 6-5: EXTERNAL FIXATION DEVICES

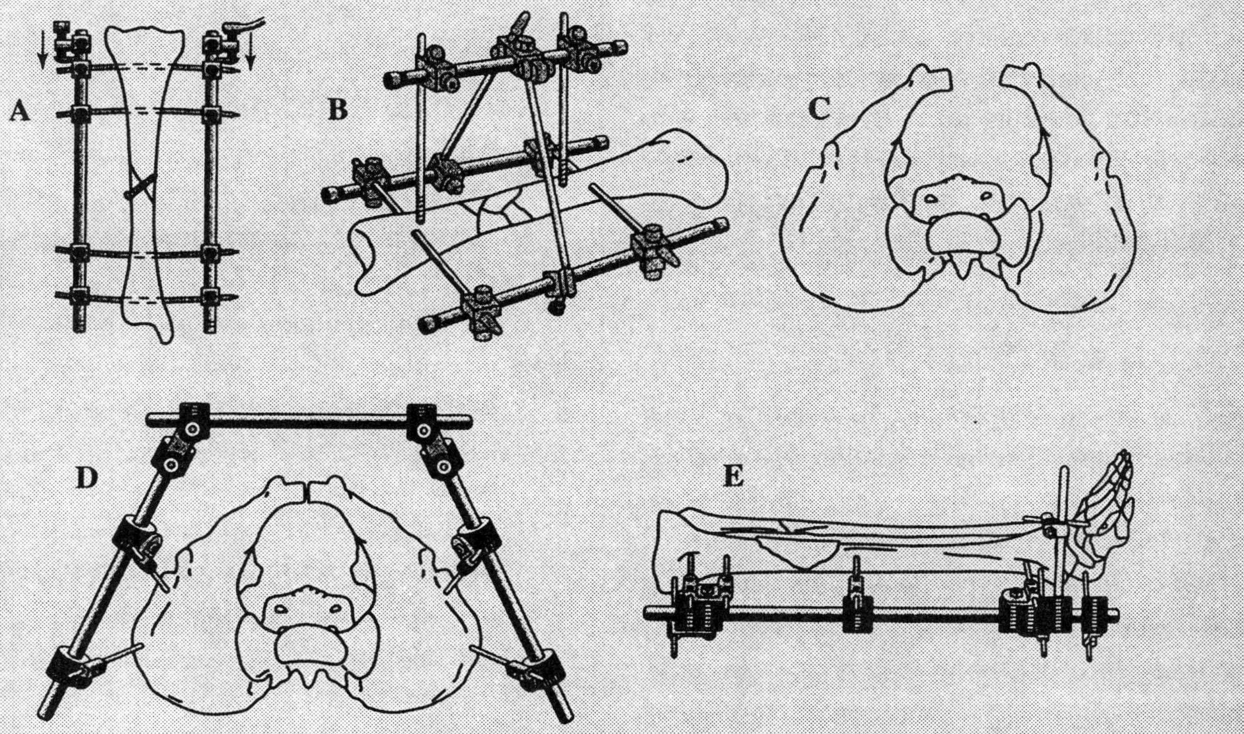

A, Tibial fracture with simple AO external fixation with lag screw at fracture site. **B,** AO (Synthes) external fixator with three-dimensional or triangular fixation of comminuted fracture of the tibia. **C,** Pelvic diastasis (dislocation). **D,** Hex-Fix™ external fixator in place, showing reduction of pelvic fracture. **E,** Hex-Fix™ external fixator used to treat tibial fracture. Immobilization of ankle and foot allows soft-tissue healing.

From Phipps, W., Sands, J., & Marek, J. (1999). *Medical Surgical Nursing: Concepts and Clinical Practice* (6th ed., p. 1922). St. Louis, MO: Mosby. Reprinted with permission from Elsevier.

ture. After the device is applied, the affected extremity is elevated to help decrease edema.

Nursing care of a patient with an external fixation device includes administering insertion site pin care during each shift and carefully inspecting the insertion sites for signs of infection. Pin care for an external device is similar to the care provided to skeletal traction pin sites and is dependent upon the physician's preferred method. The nurse never adjusts the screws on the external fixation device; only the physician can adjust the screws. Any loose pins must be reported promptly to the physician. The nurse also avoids using the device itself to move the patient's extremity. When repositioning the patient or the affected extremity, the nurse always carefully supports the extremity above and below the device.

Other nursing care includes regularly assessing the involved extremity for neurovascular impairment. The patient is encouraged to perform active exercises as tolerated to promote the return of function and strength. As the device will be left in place until the fracture is healed, many patients will be discharged home with the fixation device in place. Discharge instructions about how to care for the external fixation device are essential to prevent complications in the home setting.

SUMMARY

This chapter has described the various treatment interventions that are used when caring for patients who have experienced musculoskeletal trauma and the nursing care associated with each intervention. Good nursing care is key to preventing complications and promoting the patient's return to normal functioning.

CASE STUDY

J.H., a 35 year-old female, fractured her right tibia and fibula in a skiing accident. A long leg cast, made of plaster of Paris, is being placed on her leg to reduce and immobilize the fracture. J.H. is admitted to the orthopedic nursing unit where you are assigned to be her nurse.

Answer the following case study questions, writing your responses on a separate sheet of paper. Compare your responses to the answers that are located at the end of the chapter.

1. The newly applied cast is still damp. What precautions should be taken while the cast continues to dry? How long will it take for the cast to dry completely?

2. J.H. complains about the cast feeling "hot." How should you respond to J. H.'s concern?

3. What nursing assessments are particularly important during the first 24–48 hours following the application of the cast?

4. 8 hours after the cast application J.H. complains of increasing pain in her right leg. As you assess her right extremity, you note her right toes are pale and cool to your touch, while her left toes are warm and pink. When you passively flex her right toes, she winces in pain. From these assessment findings, what do you suspect is the problem and what should you do to intervene, if anything?

5. J.H. continues to recover and is to be discharged home with another long leg cast on her right leg. What discharge instructions should J.H. be given about cast care?

Answers to Case Study

1. The cast should be left open to air while drying. The cast should be manipulated as little as possible while it is drying; however, when it must be handled, it should be handled by the palms of the hands and not the fingers. Resting the cast on a pillow will provide some support and help prevent misshaping. J.H. should be turned every 2 hours so that a new section of the cast is exposed to the air to help facilitate drying. The patient should be cautioned not to use a blow dryer to help dry the cast as it can cause the cast to crack. Since it is made of plaster of Paris, it will take J.H.'s cast about 24–48 hours to dry completely.

2. You should tell J.H. that the feeling of heat is a normal sensation that will eventually subside as the cast dries. Instruct J.H. to keep the cast uncovered so that the heat is not allowed to build up and cause a burn.

3. Neurovascular checks are especially important during the first 24–48 hours following the application of the cast. These checks should be performed every 30 minutes during the first 4 hours following cast application. Compare assessment findings of the affected extremity to the unaffected extremity. You should check the pulse, sensation, motion, color, and temperature of the extremity distal to the cast. You should also assess for pain. Pain upon passive movement is a sign of neurovascular impairment and should be promptly reported.

4. Based upon these assessment findings, you suspect that J.H. is developing neurovascular compromise and compartment syndrome. It is essential that you intervene promptly by notifying the surgeon, elevating the extremity to the

level of the heart, and preparing to bivalve the cast. The cast can be bivalved and then spread apart to relieve pressure.

5. J.H. should be instructed to keep her right leg elevated to decrease swelling. She should be told to promptly report pain with passive movement or pain that is unrelieved by analgesics and elevation of the body part. She should also be instructed to promptly report any changes in the pulse, sensation, movement, temperature, or color of the affected body part. Additional instructions include not to insert anything down inside the cast and not to get the plaster of Paris cast wet. J.H. should also be told to inspect the cast for any drainage or hot spots and to periodically sniff the edges of the cast for any odors. Any unusual findings or elevated temperature should be reported promptly.

CHAPTER 6
Questions 29-37

29. The nurse instructing a patient in how to safely apply heat therapy to a sprained ankle should suggest

    a. applying heat therapy at night while sleeping.

    b. adjusting the temperature setting as necessary to maintain a feeling of heat.

    c. inspecting the skin following treatment for any signs of redness or tenderness.

    d. applying moisturizer to the skin before applying the heat source.

30. When a young child has experienced a femoral fracture, a cast most likely to be used to immobilize the fracture is a

    a. body jacket cast.

    b. long leg cast.

    c. cast brace.

    d. hip spica cast.

31. A nurse assessing the neurovascular status of a patient who has a fractured forearm should promptly report to the physician any

    a. pain upon passive movement.

    b. fingers that are slightly cool.

    c. mild swelling in the fingers.

    d. brisk capillary refill.

32. A nurse is inspecting a cast that was applied 3 days ago and finding an area that is warm to touch should suspect that

    a. the cast is still completing the drying process.

    b. the patient has applied pressure to that area of the cast.

    c. the fractured bone is beginning to heal.

    d. the patient is developing an infection under the cast.

33. A patient in a body cast following spinal surgery who complains of a feeling of anxiety, nausea, and abdominal pain should be treated with

    a. a change of position to side-lying.

    b. an anti-emetic and re-evaluated in 30 minutes.

    c. education about these symptoms as being related to cast syndrome.

    d. reassurance that it is normal to have indigestion with this cast.

34. Buck's traction is usually applied to

    a. repair a pelvic fracture.

    b. reduce a hip fracture prior to surgery.

    c. increase venous blood return.

    d. provide support to a fractured ankle.

35. A principle of traction is that

    a. the nurse can adjust traction weights as necessary for patient comfort.

    b. skeletal traction is never interrupted.

    c. weights must hang low to the floor to avoid injury to others.

    d. countertraction is only necessary in skeletal traction.

36. A patient with skeletal traction has an increased susceptibility to

    a. osteomyelitis.

    b. osteoporosis.

    c. osteomalacia.

    d. osteoarthritis.

37. The nursing care of a patient with an external fixation device includes

    a. maintaining the extremity in a dependent position.

    b. adjusting the screws on the device each shift.

    c. providing insertion site pin care during each shift.

    d. using the device to move the extremity.

CHAPTER 7

CARE OF PATIENTS WITH A FRACTURE

CHAPTER OBJECTIVE

After completing this chapter, the reader will be able to describe the nursing care of patients who have experienced a fracture.

LEARNING OBJECTIVES

After studying this chapter, the reader will be able to

1. discuss the various classifications of fractures.

2. specify the signs and symptoms of a fracture.

3. indicate the healing process for fractures.

4. choose the treatment modalities that are used to promote the healing of fractures.

5. indicate the general nursing care of a patient who has experienced a fracture.

6. specify the various complications associated with a fracture.

OVERVIEW

Bone fractures are one of the most commonly occurring types of musculoskeletal trauma, especially among young adult males and elderly women (Marek, 1999b). Fractures are most likely to occur as a result of a traumatic event that places undue stress on the bone, resulting in a break in the bone structure. However, some fractures occur with little or no trauma. When fractures occur in this manner, they are typically caused by an underlying disease process, such as neoplasms and osteoporosis, and are called pathological fractures. This chapter will discuss the classifications of fractures, signs and symptoms of fractures, and fracture healing. In addition, treatment modalities, the general nursing care of a patient with a fracture, and complications of fractures will be addressed.

CLASSIFICATION OF FRACTURES

Bone fractures can be classified in several different ways. One way to classify fractures is according to whether or not the skin over the fracture site has been broken (Marek, 1999b). A fracture is classified as a simple, or closed, fracture if the skin is not broken. If the skin has been broken over the fracture site, the fracture is classified as a compound, complex, or open fracture (Liddel, 2000b). Open fractures are considered contaminated and subject to infection because of the break in skin integrity (Marek, 1999b).

Another way to classify fractures is according to the location of the fracture. A fracture that occurs in a long bone may be proximal or distal, with the proximal fracture being closer to the body and the distal fracture further away from the body (Marek, 1999b). For example, a proximal fracture of the femur is located in the upper third of the femur, while a distal fracture of the femur is located in the lower third of the femur. Fractures may also be classified as complete or incomplete (Liddel, 2000b). In a complete fracture, the bone is broken through into two fragments, frequently being displaced. In an incomplete fracture, the fracture occurs on only one side of the bone.

And finally, fractures can be classified according to type (Liddel, 2000b). Figure 7-1 defines and illustrates the different types of fractures.

SIGNS AND SYMPTOMS OF A FRACTURE

The signs and symptoms of a fracture will be dependent upon the type of fracture and the location. Pain is localized, immediate and usually severe due to the soft tissue damage and muscle spasms that occur. Point tenderness over the site of the fracture may also be present. Edema develops in the fracture area as a result of bleeding; ecchymosis may eventually develop over a period of days. The patient will experience a loss of function in the involved extremity. Deformity, or abnormal bone positioning, may be present if the bone fragments are displaced or muscle spasms pull the fragments out of alignment. If the extremity is in an abnormal position, it is important that the extremity be immobilized in this position until treatment is sought. Immobilizing the fracture helps prevent further trauma and decreases pain. If it is an open fracture, the site should be covered with a sterile dressing to protect the site from further contamination. Crepitation, the grating sound produced by the movement of broken bone fragments against each other, may also be noted. The nurse should never try to deliberately elicit crepitus to assess a fracture, as the movement can produce further tissue and bone damage. If there is nerve impairment, the patient will also complain of a loss of sensation (Ruda, 2000b).

It is important for the nurse to understand that not all of the above signs and symptoms will necessarily be present in a fracture. The actual diagnosis of a fracture will be confirmed by x-ray examination (Liddel, 2000).

OVERVIEW OF THE HEALING PROCESS

The length of the fracture healing process will vary depending upon the location of the fracture site, but healing typically takes weeks to months. Factors that can impact fracture healing are listed in Table 7-1.

There are essentially six phases to the bone healing process. The first step is the development of a hematoma around the ends of the fracture, which serves to hold the fracture ends together. Secondly, the hematoma gradually gels and changes into granulation tissue. The granulation tissue, which consists of a fibrin network, provides a framework upon which osteoblasts can be deposited. In the third phase of the healing process, which usually begins about 1 week after the injury, the osteoblasts and minerals such as calcium and phosphate are deposited into this fibrin network and begin to form a callus. The callus formation can be detected on x-ray, indicating that healing of the fracture is progressing. The fourth phase of the healing process is the ossification of the callus. Calcium continues to be deposited in the callus thus providing further strengthening of the fracture site. Ossification will continue until fracture healing is complete. As ossification continues, the bone fragments are joined and consolidation occurs producing a union of the bone. In the final phase of bone healing, remodeling occurs. During the remodeling phase, excess callus is reabsorbed, and the bone becomes further strengthened and assumes the shape that it had prior to injury. At this time, weight-bearing can be gradually resumed. The stress of exercise and weighbearing will help reshape the bone and return it to normal function (Ruda, 2000b).

FIGURE 7-1: TYPES OF FRACTURES

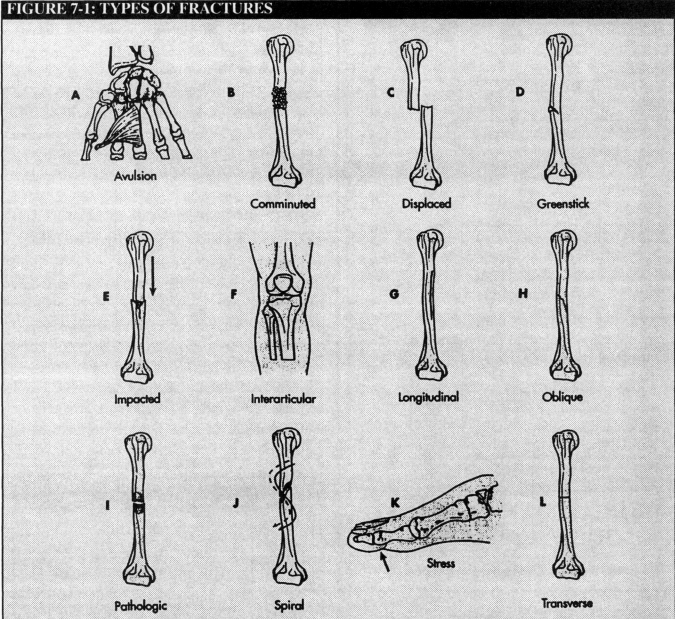

A, An avulsion is a fracture of bone resulting from the strong pulling effect of tendons or ligaments at the bone attachment. **B,** A comminuted fracture is a fracture with more than two fragments. The smaller fragments appear to be floating. **C,** A displaced (overriding) fracture involves a displaced fracture fragment that is overriding the other bone fragment. The periosteum is disrupted on both sides. **D,** A greenstick fracture is an incomplete fracture with one side splintered and the other side bent. **E,** An impacted fracture is a comminuted fracture in which more than two fragments are driven into each other. **F,** An interarticular fracture is a fracture extending to the articular surface of the bone. **G,** A longitudinal fracture is an incomplete fracture in which the fracture line runs along the longitudinal axis of the bone. The periosteum is not torn away from the bone. **H,** An oblique fracture is a fracture in which the line of the fracture extends in an oblique direction. **I,** A pathologic fracture is a spontaneous fracture at the site of a bone disease. **J,** A spiral fracture is a fracture in which the line of the fracture extends in a spiral directiTon along the shaft of the bone. **K,** A stress fracture is a fracture that occurs in normal or abnormal bone that is subject to repeated stress, such as from jogging or running. **L,** A transverse fracture is a fracture in which the line of the fracture extends across the bone shaft at a right angle to the longitudinal axis.

TABLE 7-1: FACTORS AFFECTING BONE HEALING

Favorable

Location
- Good blood supply at bone ends
- Flat bones

Minimal damage to soft tissue

Anatomic reduction possible

Effective immobilization

Weight-bearing on long bones

Unfavorable

Fragments widely separated

Fragments distracted by traction

Severely comminuted fracture

Severe damage to soft tissue

Bone loss from injury or surgical excision

Motion/rotation at fracture site as a result of inadequate fixation

Infection

Impaired blood supply to one or more bone fragments

Location
- Decreased blood supply
- Midshaft

Health behaviors such as smoking, alcohol use

From Black, J., Hawks, J., & Keene, A. (2001). *Medical-Surgical Nursing: Clinical Management of Positive Outcomes* (6th ed., p. 590). Philadelphia, PA: WB Saunders Co. Reprinted with permission from Elsevier.

MEDICAL MANAGEMENT OF A FRACTURE

The goals of the medical management of a fracture are to:

1) reduce, or realign, the fracture;

2) immobilize the fracture so that healing can occur; and

3) restore normal function to the affected area (Liddel, 2000; Ruda, 2000b).

Reduction

A fracture is reduced, or "set," to restore the bones to alignment in a normal anatomic position. A fracture can be reduced through one of two ways: 1) closed reduction or 2) open reduction. The method of reduction used to realign the bones depends upon the nature and extent of the fracture (Liddel, 2000b). For example, closed reduction is used when the bone fracture is simple and the bone fragments can be easily realigned. The reduction is accomplished by manipulation of the bone fragments, in which the physician manually realigns the bone without using surgical intervention. The patient is given an analgesic prior to the procedure and either local or general anesthesia during the manipulation. After the bone fragments are manipulated into place, a cast, traction, splint, or other device is used to immobilize the fracture for a period of time so healing can occur (Ruda, 2000b).

More complex fractures may require an open reduction to achieve realignment. In an open reduction, the patient is taken to surgery and an incision is made to allow for direct manipulation and fixation of the bone fragments (Liddel, 2000b; Ruda, 2000b). The fracture is realigned into anatomical position and held in place by the use of metal implants such as pins, wires, screws, plates, nails, or rods. Examples of these devices can be seen in Figure 7-2.

FIGURE 7-2: EXAMPLES OF INTERNAL FIXATION HARDWARE

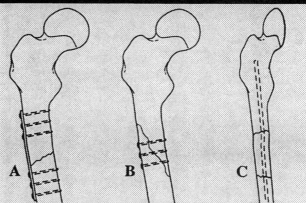

Internal fixation hardware is entirely within the body. **A,** Fixation of a short oblique fracture using a plate and screws above and below the fracture. **B,** Fixation of a long oblique fracture using screws through the fracture site. **C,** Fixation of a segmental fracture using a medullary nail.

From LeMone, Priscilla; Burke, Karen. *Medical-Surgical Nursing: Critical Thinking in Client Care,* 3rd Edition, © 2004. Reprinted by permission of Pearson Education, Inc., Upper Saddle River, NJ.

Using surgery and metal implant devices to hold a bone in alignment is referred to as an open reduction and internal fixation (ORIF). The devices may be permanent or removed after the fracture has healed depending upon the nature and location of the fracture. Patients who undergo an ORIF are at risk for developing an infection.

Immobilization

Following reduction of the fracture, the fracture will be immobilized to help promote bone healing. Immobilization of the fracture can be accomplished through the use of a cast, traction, external fixators, or internal fixators such as the metal implants described above. The length of time that the immobilization device will stay in place varies with the type and location of the fracture, the age and general condition of the patient, and the speed with which the fracture heals. Nursing care of the patient with a cast, traction, or fixation devices is described in Chapter 6 of this text.

Restoring Function

During the time that the fracture is healing, it is important for the patient to retain as much mobility and muscle tone as possible (Marek, 1999b). This will enable the patient to resume normal levels of activity more quickly after the fracture has healed, and will help prevent complications due to immobility. The physician will prescribe physical therapy for the affected part and the patient's expected level of activity. If the fracture has occurred in a lower extremity, the physician will also prescribe the amount of weight bearing that can be tolerated.

NURSING MANAGEMENT OF A PATIENT WITH A FRACTURE

The nursing management of a patient with a fracture is focused on promoting comfort, preventing complications, and achieving rehabilitation.

Promoting Comfort

Patients who have a fracture will experience acute pain related to movement of the broken bones, soft tissue swelling and injury, and muscle spasms. During the acute phase of the injury, pain control is a priority nursing goal. The nurse should assess the patient frequently for pain, using a pain scale to determine the patient's pain level (Ruda, 2000b). The nurse will administer analgesics as prescribed to control the pain. These may be narcotic or non-narcotic analgesics. The nurse should carefully evaluate the effectiveness of the analgesic, keeping in mind that unrelieved pain can be an indicator of neurovascular impairment.

In addition, muscle relaxants may also be prescribed to reduce muscle spasms. Ice compresses may be ordered in the early stages of the injury to help decrease swelling. The patient will be instructed to keep the affected part elevated and supported to help decrease swelling and pain (Ruda, 2000b). When moving and positioning the affected part, it is important that the nurse carefully and adequately support the area above and below the level of injury to minimize discomfort.

PREVENTING COMPLICATIONS

An important role of the nurse when caring for a patient with a fracture is preventing complications. The nurse plans nursing interventions that will help prevent complications and ensure early detection of any problems. One of the most serious complications that can develop with a fracture is neurovascular compromise due to edema (Marek, 1999b). When edema develops, pressure is placed on blood vessels and nerves. If not promptly relieved, the pressure can cause irreversible vessel and nerve damage. Keeping the affected extremity elevated above heart level and applying ice to prevent edema can decrease the risk of neurovascular compromise (Ruda, 2000b).

The nurse should carefully assess the patient's neurovascular status hourly during the initial phase of a fracture and immediately following reduction of the fracture, as the risk of neurovascular impairment is highest during these time periods. The components of a neurovascular assessment are listed in Table 7-2. The nurse should compare the assessment of the affected extremity with the assessment of the unaffected extremity to note any subtle differences. Any changes in the neurovascular status of an extremity should be reported promptly.

TABLE 7–2: NEUROVASCULAR ASSESSMENT
Warmth of extremity
Color of extremity
Pulses
Pain
Capillary filling time
Sensation
Voluntary movement

The nurse should also assess the patient carefully for any signs of infection. This is especially important when there has been a disruption of skin integrity as with compound fractures and open reductions. The wound should be assessed at least once a shift for signs of redness, swelling, warmth, pain, and drainage (Liddel, 2000b). Any drainage should be cultured for organisms and antibiotic therapy should be promptly initiated as appropriate. The patient's temperature should also be assessed at least every 4 hours. The patient's white blood cell count (WBC) must also be carefully monitored. Sterile asepsis is used during any dressing changes or wound care (Marek, 1999b).

If the nature of the fracture requires the patient to be immobilized for a period of time to promote healing, the nurse will develop a plan of care to prevent constipation. Ensuring a fluid intake of at least 2500 cc/day, as well as a diet high in roughage and bulk, is an important component of the care plan.

The patient should also be encouraged to remain as mobile as possible within the limits of the prescribed activity. In addition, stool softeners may be prescribed. Laxatives, suppositories, and enemas may also be necessary if constipation becomes a patient problem, but it is best to implement nursing interventions that will promote bowel elimination before constipation develops and avoid relying on the use of laxatives, suppositories, and enemas.

Renal calculi and urinary tract infections can develop in patients who are immobilized, due to increased serum calcium levels (from bone demineralization) that lead to calcium precipitation in the urine, increased urinary pH, and urinary stasis. A high fluid intake of at least 2500 cc/day is recommended to prevent urinary complications (Marek, 1999; Ruda, 2000b).

The nurse will also want to implement nursing measures to decrease venous stasis in patients who are immobilized due to a fracture. Venous stasis can lead to the development of deep vein thrombosis (DVT) and pulmonary emboli. Anti-embolic stockings or intermittent external pneumatic compression devices may be applied to the unaffected extremity to decrease venous pooling and promote venous return. Encouraging or assisting the patient to perform range of motion exercises regularly throughout the day helps prevent circulatory complications. The patient should also perform muscle setting exercises and dorsi-plantar flexion exercises with the feet hourly to encourage venous flow (Marek, 1999b).

Encouraging the patient to take slow deep breaths and cough every 2 hours. Changing positions frequently can also help prevent the development of respiratory complications, such as atelectasis and pneumonia, that can be associated with immobility. The nurse should also ensure that the patient uses incentive spirometry at least every 2 hours while immobilized to promote adequate lung expansion.

Patients who are immobilized with fractures are also at risk for developing skin breakdown in areas of bony prominences. This is particularly true of the sacrum, trochanters, heels, and the occiput of the back of the head (Fried & Fried, 2001). Scapulae and elbows are other areas that are susceptible to skin breakdown. The patient should be instructed to shift weight frequently, avoid shearing and friction of the skin tissues, and use such devices as overhead trapezes to assist with movement. If the patient is dependent upon the nursing staff for position changes, the patient should be turned at a minimum of every 2 hours and more frequently if the nurse's skin assessment uncovers evidence of redness that lasts longer than 15 minutes after pressure is relieved in an area.

Prior to discharge, the patient and the patient's family are instructed on how to prevent complications in the home setting. The nurse teaches the patient proper positioning of the affected extremity, signs and symptoms of infection, indications of neurovascular compromise, signs and symptoms of DVT, and when to notify the physician about concerns.

ACHIEVING REHABILITATION

There are several major goals of rehabilitation that the nurse should keep in mind when caring for a patient who has experienced a disabling or potentially disabling injury, such as a fracture. While this chapter is focused on the general care of the patient with a fracture, the concepts of rehabilitation that are presented here are applicable to any patient who is experiencing a prolonged period of illness or loss of function, regardless of the etiology.

One goal of rehabilitation is to restore and maintain the patient's optimal health and wellness (Hargrove & Derstine, 2001). The nurse designs a plan of care for the patient that maximizes the patient's potential in the physical, social, spiritual, and psychological dimensions of health. It is important for the nurse to focus more attention on the patient's abilities than on the patient's disabilities. Another major goal of rehabilitation is to promote

patient learning so that the patient can cope with lifestyle disruptions that might develop as a result of the injury. The nurse should also focus efforts on maintaining the patient's quality of life. Additional goals of rehabilitation include providing family-centered, culturally competent nursing care and helping the patient reintegrate into the community as a productive citizen.

Rehabilitation of the patient begins immediately after stabilization of the fracture is achieved. There are specific nursing activities that can assist the patient in regaining function. The nurse should encourage the patient to regularly perform isometric exercises and muscle setting exercises, such as quadriceps and gluteal setting exercises, to maintain muscle tone in preparation for a return to normal activities. The patient should also be encouraged to perform all activities of daily living (ADL) that can realistically be accomplished within the limitations imposed by the fracture and treatment (Marek, 1999b). Engaging in the ADL will help the patient maintain or regain functionality and will hasten the recovery phase. Range-of-motion exercises should also be performed to help maintain joint motion and function.

Assistive devices, such as crutches or walkers, may be needed to help the patient ambulate. Physical therapy may be ordered to provide gait-training and help the patient safely and correctly use these devices. The nurse reinforces all instructions for the patient and family members. The common gaits that are used with crutches are found in Table 7–3, and Figures 7–3, 7–4 and 7–5. Safety principles for crutch walking can be found in Table 7–4.

Discharge planning begins when the patient is first admitted to medical care. Depending upon the extent of the fracture and the patient's general medical condition prior to the fracture, the rehabilitation process can be a lengthy one. The patient may express many concerns, including those related to finances, loss of employment, loss of independence, changing roles within the family unit, sexuality, and

TABLE 7–3: COMMON CRUTCH GAITS

Two-Point Gait (Partial Weight Bearing)

- Left crutch and right leg advance together followed by right crutch and left leg. Repeat sequence.

Three-Point Gait (Partial or Non-Weight Bearing)

- Both crutches and the affected leg are advanced together, followed by the unaffected leg. Repeat sequence. Always advance affected leg along with both crutches, allowing the unaffected leg to provide support.

Four-Point Gait (Partial or Full Weight Bearing)

- Advance right crutch, then left foot, then left crutch, then right foot. Repeat sequence. Feet are always advanced to a position that is equal with the crutch position, never beyond.

Ascending Stairs

- Stand at foot of stairs. Patient should be instructed to place body weight on crutches. The unaffected leg is moved up to the first step, followed by the affected leg, and then the crutches. Repeat sequence. The nurse or assistant should stand beside and behind the patient on the affected side. If a hand rail is available, the patient can place both crutches in one hand and use the handrail for support as well.

Descending Stairs

- Stand at top of stairs with weight on the unaffected leg. Place crutches on first lower step. Support weight on hands and crutches, and lower the affected leg to the step with crutches. Move unaffected leg to step with crutches. Repeat sequence. The nurse or assistant can use a gait belt and stand behind the patient to provide support. If a hand rail is available, the patient can place both crutches in one hand and use the handrail for support as well.

FIGURE 7-3: FOUR-POINT ALTERNATING GAIT.

Solid feet and crutch tips show foot and crutch tip moved in each of the four phases. (Read from bottom to top.)

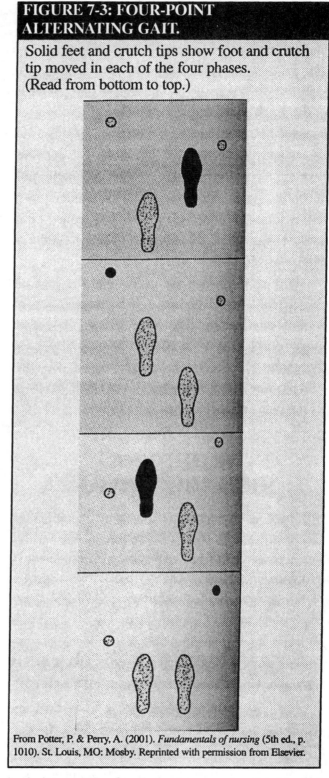

From Potter, P. & Perry, A. (2001). *Fundamentals of nursing* (5th ed., p. 1010). St. Louis, MO: Mosby. Reprinted with permission from Elsevier.

body image. The family is also very involved in the patient's recovery and may have concerns to voice as well. The nurse should provide a supportive presence, listening and encouraging the patient and family to express concerns and feelings. The nurse can

FIGURE 7-4: THREE-POINT GAIT WITH WEIGHT BORNE ON UNAFFECTED LEG.

Solid feet and crutch tips show foot and crutch tip show weight-bearing in each phase.
(Read from bottom to top.)

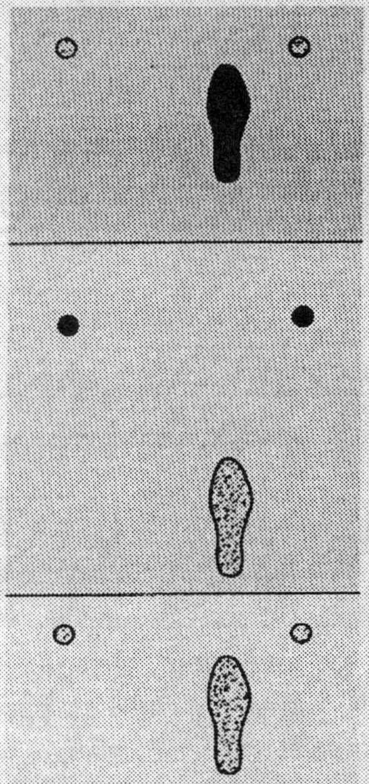

From Potter, P. & Perry, A. (2001). *Fundamentals of nursing* (5th ed., p. 1101). St. Louis, MO: Mosby. Reprinted with permission from Elsevier.

FIGURE 7-5: TWO-POINT GAIT WITH WEIGHT BORNE PARTIALLY ON EACH FOOT AND EACH CRUTCH ADVANCING WITH OPPOSING LEG.

Solid areas indicate leg and crutch tips bearing weight. (Read from bottom to top.)

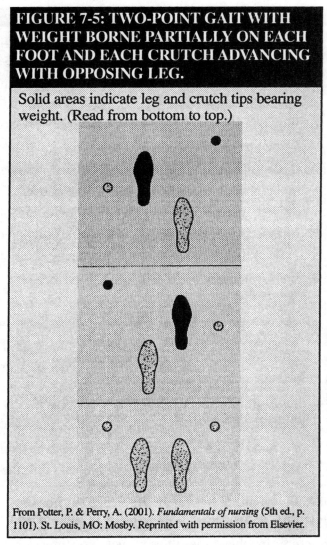

From Potter, P. & Perry, A. (2001). *Fundamentals of nursing* (5th ed., p. 1101). St. Louis, MO: Mosby. Reprinted with permission from Elsevier.

act as a resource and referral agent to address any psychosocial concerns of the patient or family members. The nurse can also help the patient and family access any support services and acquire any assistive devices that may be required when the patient returns home. How to safely use assistive devices and how to avoid the hazards of immobility are two important patient education topics that the nurse should include in the patient's education plan.

COMPLICATIONS OF A FRACTURE

Most fractures will heal without complication. There are, however, several complications that can develop as a result of a fracture, and the nurse needs to be knowledgeable about these potential complications and assess the patient according-

ly. Early detection of complications can be life-saving or prevent permanent disability. Some complications, such as shock, infection, fat embolism syndrome, and compartment syndrome, develop in the earlier phases of injury and treatment. Other complications, such as delayed union or nonunion of the fracture, develop later in the healing process. The complications that are addressed in the following discussion include hypovolemic shock, fat embolism syndrome, pulmonary embolism, compartment syndrome, infection, and delayed union or nonunion of the bone.

Hypovolemic Shock

Bone is very vascular, and a fracture can lead to internal or external hemorrhage. Hypovolemic shock can develop if the patient loses large quanti-

TABLE 7–4: SAFETY PRINCIPLES FOR CRUTCH WALKING

1. Patient should regularly perform upper-body strengthening exercises in preparation for crutch use.

2. Crutches should be adjusted to correctly fit the patient. (With the patient standing, position the crutches about 5 inches lateral on either side of the patient and about 5 inches in front of the client. The crutch pad should fit approximately 2 inches below the axilla and the hands should rest on the hand grips in a position that allows 30 degrees of flexion in the elbows).

3. Patient should wear comfortable, firm, low-heeled walking shoes.

4. Gait belt should be place around the waist if balance and stability are questionable. When assisting patient to ambulate with crutches, stand slightly behind and to the affected side of the patient with one hand positioned on the gait belt. Do not pull on the patient, as this can affect balance.

5. Inspect tips of crutches for wear at frequent intervals.

6. Always inspect nuts and bolts on crutches prior to use to ensure tightness.

7. Caution patient not to lean on axilla crutch pad, as this can lead to brachial nerve plexus pressure.

8. If patient complains of tingling in hands and arms, which is indicative of brachial nerve pressure, inspect the crutches for appropriate fit and observe patient's use of crutches.

9. When sitting in a chair, the patient advances to the chair, turns around, and carefully backs up to the chair until the unaffected leg touches the chair. Both crutches are then placed in the hand of the unaffected side, and the patient carefully reaches for the arm or seat of the chair with the hand on the affected side, and carefully lowers self to the chair, moving the affected leg forward. To get up from the chair, the crutches are positioned on the unaffected side of the patient and used to push the patient up, while the patient uses the hand on the affected side to help push up from the chair. The unaffected leg bears the weight while the patient assumes an upright position, and then the crutches are transferred to the correct standing position.

ties of blood immediately following a fracture (Stewart, 2000). Shock is more likely to occur if the fracture involves the thorax, pelvis, spine, or extremities, especially the femur. Patients experiencing a fracture of this type should be closely assessed for developing shock. Treatment of hypovolemic shock consists of restoring blood volume with rapid infusion of intravenous fluids, controlling the patient's pain, and splinting and minimizing movement of the fracture (Schoen, 2000).

Fat Embolism Syndrome

Fat Embolism Syndrome (FES) is a potentially fatal complication of fractures. FES most commonly occurs in patients who have experienced a fracture of the femur, tibia, pelvis, or multiple fractures (Marek, 1999b). It usually develops within the first 24–48 hours after injury. After a fracture, it is theorized that fat globules are released from the bone

marrow and enter into the patient's bloodstream, where the emboli travel to the lungs and become lodged in pulmonary capillaries (Ruda, 2000b). Another theory is that catecholamines are released due to the trauma, leading to an alteration in lipid stability that results in the development of fat globules that enter the bloodstream (Schoen, 2000).

The signs and symptoms of FES can be subtle at first and are related to interference with oxygen exchange (hypoxia). Signs and symptoms that include altered mental status, personality changes, irritability, restlessness, or agitation are frequently the presenting indicators of FES. The patient may also express a feeling of impending doom. The nurse should suspect FES and intervene promptly in any patient with a fracture who suddenly exhibits these symptoms. It is extremely important that the symptoms of FES be detected early to increase the patient's chances of survival. FES is a medical emergency that requires prompt intervention. As FES progresses, signs of tachypnea, dyspnea, tachycardia, fever, and a petechial rash on the neck, axilla, chest, and conjunctiva may develop and progress. The patient may also complain of chest pain, and skin color can range from pale to cyanotic. FES progresses rapidly, and the patient may become comatose (Marek, 1999b; Ruda, 2000b). Death can result.

FES is best treated by prevention. Minimal manipulation of a fracture and stabilization as soon as possible after the injury are important. Early detection of FES is an important nursing intervention. Treatment of FES is supportive, with the goal of preventing adult respiratory distress syndrome and respiratory failure. If FES is suspected, arterial blood gases will be obtained. In FES, the PaO2 is decreased and the PCO2 is increased (Marek, 1999b). Chest x-rays will show a snowstorm infiltrate (Ruda, 2000b).

Oxygen therapy in high concentrations is administered to patients with FES, and the patient is placed in a high Fowler's position. Mechanical ventilation with positive end-expiratory pressure may also be needed to support respiratory functioning (Liddel, 2000b).

Pulmonary Embolism

Pulmonary embolism (PE) is a common cause of death in patients who have experienced an orthopedic injury or surgery in the lower extremities. The cause of a PE is likely to be a deep vein thrombosis that breaks off and travels through the circulation until it lodges in a pulmonary artery. The lodged embolus causes an obstruction of blood flow to the affected areas of the lung, leading to an infarction of lung tissue. Many patients who experience a PE are asymptomatic; the patient with a massive PE suddenly experiences an onset of severe dyspnea, cyanosis, substernal chest pain, tachycardia, shock, and, in some cases, sudden death (Schoen, 2000). Patients with less massive PE typically develop tachycardia, dyspnea, tachypnea, hemoptysis, rales,

and a cough. The patient may complain of pleuritic chest pain, develop a fever, and appear anxious. The diagnosis of PE may confirmed by a chest x-ray, ventilation-perfusion scan, and arterial blood gases.

Treatment of PE consists of placing the patient in a semi-Fowler's position, administering oxygen, monitoring vital signs, and administering anticoagulant therapy. Prevention of PE, however, is the best treatment. The nurse should take care to implement nursing interventions that promote venous return and prevent venous stasis. Such interventions include using anti-embolus stockings, using intermittent external pneumatic compression devices, encouraging leg and ankle exercises, and maintaining the patient's hydration.

Compartment Syndrome

Compartment syndrome is a complication that develops when the circulation to an upper or lower extremity area is compromised, due to tissue swelling within the closed compartment of a muscle fascial sheath. The swelling can result from serious tissue trauma or the application of external devices such as casts, splints, or constricting dressings. The tissue swelling causes an increase of pressure and compression within the compartment. As the pressure increases, the blood vessels become constricted, resulting in a lack of circulation to the tissues. Ischemia develops. If the pressure is not relieved promptly, the compression and ischemia will ultimately lead to the destruction of muscle tissue and nerve damage. In this case, the patient will experience irreversible muscle and nerve damage resulting in muscle atrophy, contractures, and loss of function (Ruda, 2000b). The onset of permanent damage is quick, frequently developing within 4 to 12 hours of the onset of ischemia (Marek, 1999b).

Certain types of fractures are more likely to lead to the development of compartment syndrome. Fractures of the proximal tibia and the distal humerus are the two most common fractures to lead to the development of compartment syndrome

(Ruda, 2000b). Although less common, other areas that can develop compartment syndrome include the hand, shoulder, thigh, and buttocks (Schoen, 2000).

Signs and symptoms of compartment syndrome include pain that is severe, progressive, and unrelieved by analgesics. This is the most common sign, and it is essential that the nurse report such a finding immediately to the physician so that prompt intervention can occur. Additional signs and symptoms include pain upon passive movement of extremity or digits, pallor, paresthesia, diminished or absent pulses, and coolness in the extremity. Absent pulses are a late sign indicating that severe circulatory compromise has occurred (Ruda, 2000b).

Intervention must be prompt when compartment syndrome is suspected. Any restricting devices such as casts, splints, or dressings must be split, loosened, or removed. Do not apply ice or elevate the extremity above the level of the heart, as these actions may further impair circulation. If removing restrictive devices does not lessen the pressure, then the physician will perform a fasciotomy. An incision is made into the fascia to relieve pressure. This incision will be left open until pressure within the compartment has been resolved (Liddel, 2000b). During this time, the wound is covered with moist, sterile dressings.

Infection

Infection is a common complication of open fractures. Infection may also develop as a result of surgical intervention with internal fixation of a fracture or when external devices are used to stabilize a fracture. Prevention of infection is the best treatment. Once an infection develops in the bone, the resulting osteomyelitis may be resistant to treatment and require long-term care. Infection can also lead to delayed union or nonunion of the fracture (Schoen, 2000). Antibiotic therapy is used to treat infections.

Delayed Union or Nonunion

Occasionally fractures will be slow to heal or will not heal at all. Delayed union refers to a situation where the bone is healing, but it is taking a longer period of time than anticipated. Frequently delayed union is caused by the presence of an infection. It may also be caused by inadequate stabilization of the fracture or poor blood supply. When the underlying cause of the delayed union is treated, the fracture eventually heals (Schoen, 2000).

In a nonunion, the fracture displays no signs of healing. The bone fragments of the fracture remain separated. Nonunion can occur because of infection, poor circulation, inadequate stabilization, a reduction of fracture that resulted in a bone gap between fragments, or the presence of tissue or muscle trapped between the bone ends. Poor nutrition may also cause a nonunion (Schoen, 2000). The treatment for a nonunion is a bone graft. The bone graft may either be an allograft (from another donor) or an autograft (from the patient). The bone graft stimulates bone growth and eventual healing of the fracture. Following a bone graft, the fracture must remain immobilized with no weight bearing throughout the entire healing period. Another treatment for nonunion is the use of electrical stimulation. Electrical impulses are applied to the nonunion area to stimulate bone growth. This treatment may take up to 6 months or more to produce a union (Liddel, 2000).

SUMMARY

This chapter discussed the classifications of fractures, signs and symptoms of fractures, and fracture healing. In addition, treatment modalities, the general nursing care of a patient with a fracture, and complications of fractures were addressed. Careful assessment by the nurse, with prompt intervention when potential complications are identified, is essential to the delivery of safe nursing care in the patient who has experienced a fracture. It is also important for the nurse to understand the process of fracture healing and union so that the appropriate therapeutic interventions can be provided in a timely manner to promote healing. Improper immobilization, poor nutrition, poor circulation, and infection can all impact the healing process. The nurse's awareness of these factors and implementation of nursing actions to prevent complications will support the healing process and result in a positive outcome for the patient.

EXAM QUESTIONS

CHAPTER 7
Questions 38-50

38. Fractures that occur as a result of an underlying disease process are called

    a. open fractures.

    b. comminuted fractures.

    c. pathological fractures.

    d. complex fractures.

39. A bone that has been broken into several fragments is called a

    a. compound fracture.

    b. spiral fracture.

    c. transverse fracture.

    d. comminuted fracture.

40. One sign or symptom of a fracture is

    a. lengthened extremity.

    b. loss of function.

    c. contracture.

    d. referred pain.

41. A person typically can begin resuming weight-bearing activities during the

    a. callus formation phase of bone healing.

    b. remodeling phase of bone healing.

    c. ossification phase of bone healing.

    d. granulation tissue formation phase of bone healing.

42. The process of restoring fractured bones to their normal anatomical alignment is called

    a. reduction.

    b. fixation.

    c. traction.

    d. realignment.

43. An open reduction and internal fixation of a fractured femur involves

    a. the insertion of metal implant devices into the femur.

    b. the application of skin traction.

    c. total bedrest for 1 week following the procedure.

    d. a bone graft to stimulate healing.

44. To reduce swelling in an extremity with a newly sustained fracture, the patient should be instructed to

    a. apply a heating pad to the extremity.

    b. do quadriceps setting exercises daily.

    c. elevate the extremity.

    d. keep the extremity immobilized.

45. One of the most serious complications that can develop in the early stages of a fracture is

    a. an infection.

    b. neurovascular compromise.

    c. a contracture.

    d. nonunion.

46. Following a fracture, rehabilitation of the patient will begin

    a. immediately upon stabilization of the fracture.

    b. when the patient's pain is decreased.

    c. approximately 4 weeks after the bone begins healing.

    d. when the potential for complications has decreased.

47. One of the earliest indicators of fat embolism syndrome (FES) may be

    a. dyspnea.

    b. petechial rash.

    c. fever.

    d. altered mental status.

48. The nurse who suspects a patient with a fracture of the tibia may be developing fat embolism syndrome (FES) should

    a. immediately place the patient in a supine position.

    b. promptly notify the physician of the patient's symptoms.

    c. carefully reassess the patient's condition hourly.

    d. monitor the patient closely for the development of chest pain.

49. The nurse who suspects that a patient with a fractured tibia has developed compartment syndrome should

    a. elevate the extremity immediately above the heart level.

    b. loosen or remove any restrictive devices on the extremity.

    c. apply ice packs to the lower portion of the extremity.

    d. administer opioid analgesics to decrease pain.

50. Four weeks after casting a fractured humerus, an x-ray reveals that there has been no healing at the fracture site, a complication called

    a. malunion.

    b. delayed union.

    c. nonunion.

    d. unstable union.

CHAPTER 8

CARE OF PATIENTS WITH SPECIFIC FRACTURES

CHAPTER OBJECTIVE

After completing this chapter, the reader will be able to describe the medical management and nursing care of patients who have experienced a fracture of the upper extremity or lower extremity. Fractures of the clavicle, pelvis, and spine will also be addressed.

LEARNING OBJECTIVES

After studying this chapter, the reader will be able to

1. indicate the medical management of the patient who has experienced a fracture of the clavicle, upper extremity, pelvis, spine, or lower extremity.

2. specify the nursing care of the patient who has experienced a fracture of the clavicle, upper extremity, pelvis, spine, or lower extremity.

3. indicate the principles of rehabilitation for a patient who has experienced a fracture of the clavicle, upper extremity, pelvis, spine, or lower extremity.

OVERVIEW

The medical management and nursing care of a patient who has experienced a fracture will vary depending upon the type and location of the fracture. The nurse must have an understanding of the patient needs related to the specific fracture to provide safe and competent nursing care. This chapter will discuss the care of patients who have experienced fractures of the clavicle, upper extremity, pelvis, spine, or lower extremity. Special emphasis will be placed on the rehabilitation process and assisting the patient to avoid complications and regain full function following a fracture.

FRACTURE OF THE CLAVICLE

Fractures of the clavicle, or collarbone, are common fractures, especially in children. The most likely cause of a clavicle fracture is a direct blow to the shoulder or a fall where the person tries to break the fall with an extended arm (Schoen, 2000). Contact sports are likely causes of clavicle fractures.

A patient who has experienced a fractured clavicle experiences pain and slumps the shoulders forward. The patient usually holds the arm to minimize movement and protect the clavicle. Treatment of the fracture involves realignment and immobilization of the clavicle using a clavicular strap that holds the shoulders back in place (see Figure 8–1). If the fracture has occurred in the distal third of the clavicle and is not displaced, the only treatment may be a sling that serves to immobilize the arm (Liddel, 2000b).

Clavicular fractures usually heal without complication within about 6 weeks. During the healing time, the patient is instructed by the nurse not to lift the arm

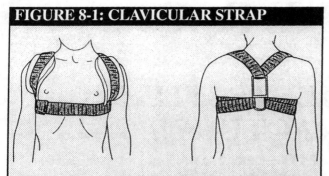

FIGURE 8-1: CLAVICULAR STRAP

Immobilization is accomplished with a clavicular strap.

From LeMone, Priscilla; Burke, Karen. *Medical-Surgical Nursing: Critical Thinking in Client Care*, 3rd Edition, © 2004. Reprinted by permission of Pearson Education, Inc., Upper Saddle River, NJ.

above shoulder level. The patient is encouraged, however, to continue exercising the fingers, wrist, and elbow to prevent loss of function. Complications, if they do occur, are related to brachial nerve damage, subclavian artery or vein damage, or malunion of the bone ends (Liddel, 2000b).

FRACTURE OF THE UPPER EXTREMITY

Fractures of the upper extremity include fractures of the humerus, ulna, radius, wrist, and hand. Each of these fracture locations will be briefly discussed, including medical management and nursing care appropriate for the specific location.

Humerus

Humerus fractures may occur proximally (near the shoulder), distally (near the elbow), or in the shaft of the humerus. Humerus fractures are caused either by a direct blow to the arm or indirectly by the person trying to break a fall with an outstretched arm. Fractures of the humerus usually heal within 6–10 weeks.

A fractured humeral shaft is one of the most common fractures and usually heals rapidly without complication. Because of the relatively small size of the arm muscles, the fractured bone ends typically remain aligned and do not override each other. This maintenance of alignment makes reduction of the fracture easier to achieve and promotes healing. Most humeral shaft fractures can be reduced through closed manipulation and the placement of a functional cast. A functional cast involves the placement of a plastic splint device around the patient's upper arm, while a sling supports the lower arm. The functional cast provides minimal immobilization of the humerus, while allowing gravity to maintain alignment of the fracture. The advantage of a functional cast is that it promotes movement of the shoulder, elbow joint, and wrist, thus helping to prevent loss of function of these joints while the fracture heals (Schoen, 2000).

A hanging arm cast, which provides more immobilization and is allowed to hang down to promote the use of gravity, may also be used to treat humeral fractures. Hanging arm casts are more likely to be used for displaced fractures, especially oblique or spiral fractures, which have caused shortening in the extremity. Hanging casts provide additional "pull" or traction on the arm to maintain alignment of the fracture due to their weight. Occasionally, an open reduction and internal fixation surgical procedure may be necessary to reduce the fracture and hold the bone ends in alignment with screws, plates, or pins. The two most common complications of humeral shaft fractures are nonunion and radial nerve damage (Schoen, 2000).

A fracture of the proximal humerus, which is near the shoulder, usually occurs in or near the surgical or anatomical neck of the humerus. A common type of proximal humerus fracture is the impacted fracture that occurs when the person tries to break a fall with an outstretched arm. This type of fracture is especially common in the elderly. An impacted fracture is not displaced and usually heals without difficulty, requiring only a sling to support the arm while the fracture heals. Patients are encouraged to do pendulum exercises as tolerated during the healing period to prevent shoulder stiffness and maintain functionality. If the fracture is displaced, the distal fragment of the fracture is usually pulled upward to override the proximal fragment. A closed or open reduction will be necessary to regain alignment (Schoen, 2000). Complications related to the fracture of the proximal humerus include damage to the nerves and blood vessels in the area of injury (Liddel, 2000b).

Fractures of the distal humerus are located near the elbow joint. This type of fracture is most common in children and the elderly. To treat a fracture of a distal humerus, the fracture is reduced through either closed or open reduction, and a cast is placed on the arm with the elbow placed in 45–90 degrees of flexion to maintain bone alignment. If the fracture was displaced, side-arm traction may be necessary to maintain alignment (see Figure 8–2). Distal humerus fractures may cause injury to the ulnar, radial, or median nerves. These fractures are particularly susceptible to the development of compartment syndrome which, if not treated promptly, can result in a Volkmann's ischemic contracture of the hand and arm (Schoen, 2000). Figure 8–3 shows a picture of Volkmann's contracture.

FIGURE 8-2: LATERAL ARM IMMOBILIZATION

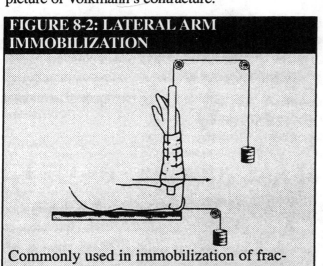

Commonly used in immobilization of fractures and dislocations of the upper arm and shoulder.
Inspect the pin site and perform pin site care according to hospital policy. Assess neurovascular status.

From Lewis, S., Heitkemper, M., & Dirksen, S. (2000). *Medical-surgical nursing: Assessment and management of clinical problems* (5th ed., p. 1775). St. Louis: Mosby. Reprinted with permission from Elsevier.

FIGURE 8-3: VOLKMANN'S ISCHEMIC CONTRACTURE.

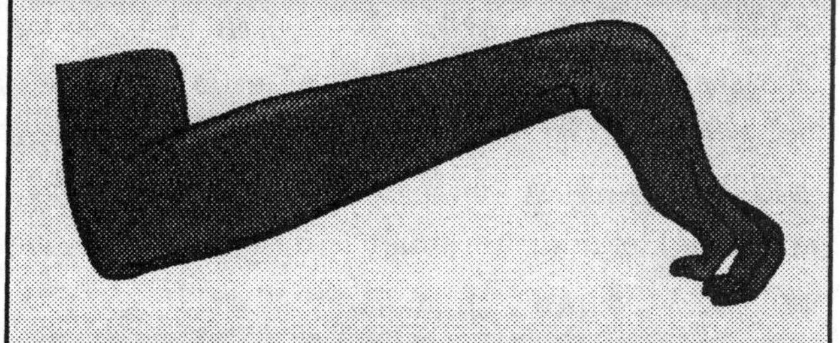

From Phipps, W., Sands, J., & Marek, J. (1999). *Medical surgical nursing: Concepts and clinical practice* (6th ed., p. 1935). St. Louis, MO: Mosby. Reprinted with permission from Elsevier.

Nursing care of the patient with a fractured humerus is focused on pain relief, prevention or early detection of complications, and maintenance of joint function in the affected arm. It will be important for the nurse to encourage or assist the patient to perform activities of daily living within his or her ability and to do range-of-motion exercises of all uninvolved joints at least every 4 hours during waking hours. The affected extremity is exercised as ordered by the physician (Schoen, 2000).

Radius and Ulna

Fractures of the forearm are common, with fractures of the radius being most common. While the radius alone may be fractured, it is rare for the ulna alone to be fractured. If the ulna is fractured, it is likely that the radius has suffered a fracture as well. When either the radius or ulna is fractured, the most common concern is displacement of the fractures, especially in adults. Because the major movements of the forearm are supination and pronation, when reducing the fractures and achieving alignment care must be given to align the bone ends such that the functions of supination and pronation will be preserved. The pull of the various muscles in the forearm can make it difficult for this alignment to be achieved through closed reduction alone, especially in adults (Schoen, 2000).

If the fracture of the radius and/or ulna is not displaced, a closed reduction will be performed and a long arm cast applied. If the fracture is displaced, an open reduction will be necessary along with internal fixation of the bone ends (Liddel, 2000b). Fractures that have occurred above the pronator *radii teres* will require that the forearm be placed in a supine position to properly align the bone ends. Fractures that have occurred below the pronator *radii teres* will require that the forearm be placed in a pronated position to achieve alignment. Casts are applied to the arm to maintain the healing position (Schoen, 2000).

Fractures of the radius and ulna usually require immobilization for approximately 12 weeks. Nursing care immediately following reduction of the fracture include keeping the arm elevated to decrease edema. In addition, patients are encouraged to flex and extend fingers of the affected arm frequently to encourage circulation and decrease edema. Neurovascular checks, which include an assessment of the affected extremity's circulation, sensation, and movement, are performed frequently to detect early changes that may indicate neurovascular compromise (Liddel, 2000b). If the patient is discharged home immediately following placement of a cast on a nondisplaced fracture, it is important that the nurse provide discharge teaching that emphasizes keeping the arm elevated, assessing the neurovascular status of the affected arm, performing cast care, and achieving pain control. It is also important to teach the patient how to maintain function of the shoulder in the affected arm. Even though the arm is immobilized by a cast, shoulder exercises are necessary to avoid loss of function in the shoulder area.

Wrist and Hand

The most common fracture of the wrist is a fracture of the distal radius known as a Colles' fracture. These fractures are commonly seen in elderly women who have osteoporosis and have experienced a fall on an outstretched, dorsiflexed hand. Upon examination the wrist will look swollen, deformed and deviate towards the radius. The patient will complain of pain and may experience numbness as well (Liddel, 2000b). Most Colles' fractures can be treated with closed manipulation

and the placement of a cast. It is important that the patient keep the hand elevated at heart level the first couple of days following the injury to reduce swelling in the fingers (Schoen, 2000). To prevent stiffness and loss of function in fingers and shoulder, the patient is taught active exercises that will help keep swelling to a minimum and retain function. One potential complication of a Colles' fracture is median nerve damage. The nurse can assess for median nerve damage by checking the patient's thumb opposition to the little finger and by pricking the distal surface of the index finger to test sensation (Liddel, 2000b).

Fractures of the hand can be highly variable, ranging from simple, nondisplaced fractures of the fingers to traumatic injuries that require extensive reconstruction. For nondisplaced closed fractures of the hand, closed reduction and cast immobilization for 6-12 weeks will likely be the treatment of choice. Most hand fractures heal rapidly because of the good blood supply to the area (Schoen, 2000). Fractures that are displaced or open may require an open reduction with the insertion of pins or wires. Nursing care following reduction of the fracture includes frequent neurovascular checks and keeping the hand elevated to decrease edema. Range of motion exercises, as appropriate, will be encouraged to maintain hand functionality.

FRACTURE OF THE PELVIS

The most likely cause of a pelvic fracture is a motor vehicle accident. Pelvic fractures can result in very serious injuries. Many patients who experience pelvic fractures also suffer additional trauma at the time of the injury. Pelvic fractures themselves can cause significant injury to the organs that lie in the immediate area, such as the bladder and colon. Due to the vascularity of the area, pelvic fractures are also associated with a high risk of hemorrhage and hypovolemic shock, which can be life-threatening if not detected and treated early. Patients who experience a pelvic fracture are also susceptible to complications during the rehabilitation phase. These complications include fat emboli, deep vein thrombosis, pulmonary emboli, and infection. To avoid these complications a goal of treatment will be to stabilize the fracture and encourage early mobility.

Clinical indications of a pelvic fracture include swelling, ecchymosis, unusual movement in the pelvic area, and tenderness (Ruda, 2000b). In addition, the patient may experience numbness and tingling in the pubic area and upper thighs. The patient will also have difficulty bearing weight due to the pain (Liddel, 2000b). Pelvic fractures may be either stable or unstable. Figure 8–4 depicts the various types of stable pelvic fractures.

FIGURE 8-4: EXAMPLE OF STABLE PELVIC FRACTURES

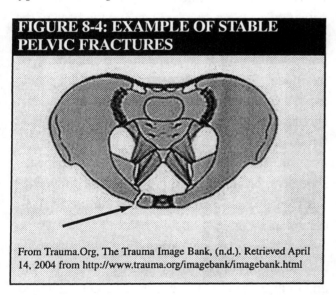

From Trauma.Org, The Trauma Image Bank, (n.d.). Retrieved April 14, 2004 from http://www.trauma.org/imagebank/imagebank.html

Management of pelvic fractures includes the early detection of complications. Hemorrhage and the potential for hypovolemic shock are significant clinical concerns immediately post-injury, so the patient will be monitored closely for signs of bleeding. Another clinical concern is adequate nerve and blood supply to both lower extremities, so frequent neurovascular checks of the lower extremities are essential. Patients must also be closely examined for injury to the colon, bladder, and urinary tract, and they will likely undergo a series of x-rays or CT scans to detect injury to underlying abdominal structures.

Treatment of the fracture itself will depend upon the severity of the injury. If the patient has a stable fracture of the pelvis, it is possible that the fracture can be treated with bed rest for a prescribed period of time (Ruda, 2000b). Pelvic fractures can heal quickly due to the vascular nature of the area, so healing may occur within 6 weeks. Unstable pelvic fractures will require either an open reduction and internal fixation or an external fixation to promote stabilization of the fracture and early mobility. Figure 8–5 depicts illustrations of unstable pelvic fractures. Skeletal traction may also be necessary to maintain alignment.

FIGURE 8-5: EXAMPLE OF UNSTABLE PELVIC FRACTURES

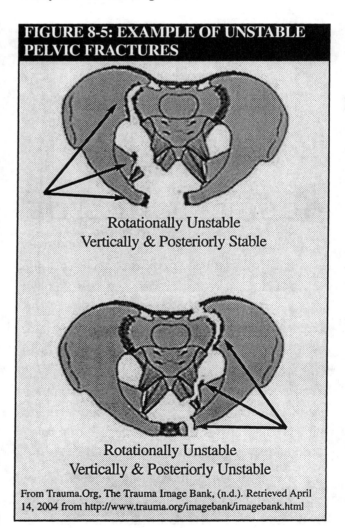

Rotationally Unstable
Vertically & Posteriorly Stable

Rotationally Unstable
Vertically & Posteriorly Unstable

From Trauma.Org, The Trauma Image Bank, (n.d.). Retrieved April 14, 2004 from http://www.trauma.org/imagebank/imagebank.html

During the time the patient is on bedrest, it is essential that the nurse encourage range of motion to all unaffected joints, as well as ankle pumps and leg exercises so that mobility and circulation can be maintained and the hazards of immobility avoided. Muscle setting exercises, such as gluteal and quadriceps setting, help maintain muscle tone and improve circulation. Elastic compression stockings and sequential compression devices may also be used to decrease venous stasis. The patient should be turned to the side only as ordered by the physician. If turning is allowed, the patient is typically tilted to the side at approximately 45 degrees, and log rolling will be used to maintain alignment (Schoen, 2000). The patient should be repositioned every 2 hours.

Adequate fluid and nutritional intake, pain control, skin care, coughing, and deep breathing are all aspects of the nursing care plan. Urinary output and bowel function are closely monitored as well. As the patient recovers, ambulation is gradually resumed with the aid of a walker or crutches to assist with weight bearing (Liddel, 2000b).

FRACTURE OF THE SPINE

Fractures of the spine are most commonly caused by traumatic accidents such as motor vehicle accidents, sports injuries, and falls. In older individuals, osteoporosis is a common cause of vertebral fractures. Metastatic bone cancer can also lead to pathological fractures of the spine. The area of the spine that is most susceptible to fracture is the T12 to L2 area (Liddel, 2000b). The most common type of vertebral fracture is a compression fracture which is caused by an excessive vertical load being placed on the spine (Ruda, 2000b).

Fractures of the spine may be either stable or unstable. Most spinal fractures are stable fractures that do not cause damage to the spinal cord. An unstable fracture, in which there is an actual displacement of the fracture, can result in spinal cord

injury and possibly permanent disability. This discussion is focused on stable spinal fractures.

Patients who have experienced a spinal fracture will complain of acute pain in the area of the injury accompanied by paravertebral muscle spasms. The patient experiences increased pain upon weight-bearing and movement. A stable spinal fracture does not produce any neurological deficits. If the patient experiences any neurological deficits, the patient is likely to require immediate surgery to reduce the pressure being placed on the spinal cord and prevent further injury (Liddel, 2000b).

All patients with a suspected spinal fracture should be treated as if the fracture is unstable until proven otherwise with x-rays. The majority of spinal fractures can be treated conservatively, with the patient being placed on bed rest and the head of the bed elevated no more than 30 degrees. The main goal of treatment is to maintain the spine in good alignment while healing occurs. The patient should avoid an upright position during this acute phase and should also avoid twisting the back when being turned in bed. The nurse will assist the patient to turn using the log rolling technique so that the patient's shoulders, back, and hips are all turned simultaneously in one unit. Analgesics are administered to control pain. In addition to bedrest, heat may be applied to help relieve muscle spasms. In some instances, skin traction may also be applied to help immobilize the fracture, decrease compression and muscle spasms, and decrease pain (Ruda, 2000b).

The nurse should assess the patient's neurovascular status frequently to detect any neurological changes. Bladder and bowel control should also be assessed. Any difficulty in controlling bowel or bladder function or any changes in sensation or movement of the extremities should be immediately reported to the physician (Ruda, 2000b).

As the pain decreases, the patient will be allowed to gradually resume activity. An orthotic device (back brace) will be fitted to the patient so that the patient can keep the spine in alignment when ambulating. If the spinal fracture is in the cervical area, the patient may be fitted with a collar or halo vest (see Figure 8–6) to limit movement of the cervical spine. The patient is discharged home when able to safely ambulate and care for the orthotic device (Ruda, 2000b).

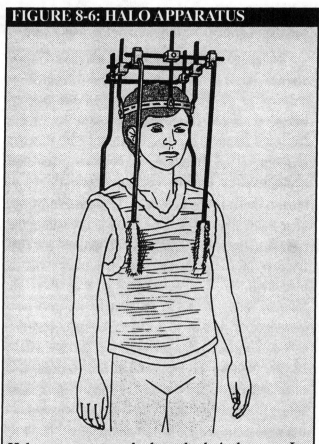

FIGURE 8-6: HALO APPARATUS

Halo apparatus attached to a body jacket cast. It may also be attached to a brace. A halo vest can be used in treatment of a cervical spine injury or following cervical spine surgery.

From Lewis, S., Heitkemper, M., & Dirksen, S. (2000). *Medical-surgical nursing: Assessment and management of clinical problems* (5th ed., p. 1794). St. Louis, MO: Mosby. Reprinted with permission from Elsevier.

FRACTURE OF THE LOWER EXTREMITY

Fractures of the lower extremity involve the femur, tibia, and fibula. Each of these fracture locations will be briefly discussed, including medical management and nursing care appropriate for the specific location.

Femur

Fractures of the femur can occur in the neck of the femur or in the proximal, midshaft, or distal sections (see Figure 8–7). This discussion on femoral fractures will focus on femoral shaft fractures that occur either proximally, midshaft, or distally. Fractures of the femoral neck will be discussed in Chapter 9, on care of the patient with a hip fracture. Treatment will vary depending upon the type of femoral fracture the patient has experienced.

Fracturing a femur in an adult individual requires a significant amount of force. This force is usually the result of a traumatic event such as a motor vehicle accident, fall, or sports accident. Young adults are typically the ones who experience a fractured femur. Because of the amount of force necessary to fracture a femur, it is quite likely that the patient will also experience soft tissue injuries and other trauma as well.

The clinical manifestations of a fractured femoral shaft include acute pain, swelling, deformity in the thigh, angulation, shortening of the extremity due to muscle pull, and an inability to move the hip or knee (Liddel, 2000b; Ruda, 2000b). Patients who have a fractured femur must be closely assessed for hemorrhage, which can result from soft tissue damage and the subsequent onset of hypovolemic shock. The neurovascular status of the affected extremity also needs to be closely assessed at frequent intervals. The nurse should compare the neurovascular assessment of the affected leg to the unaffected leg to note any differences. Peripheral pulses can be checked with a Doppler device (Stewart, 2000). Initial treatment of a fractured femur is focused on immobilizing the fracture to prevent further injury and minimize hemorrhaging. In addition the fracture is manipulated as little as necessary to reduce the chances of a fat embolism. Intravenous fluids will be administered to replace blood volume loss and administer any antibiotic therapy for open fractures (Stewart, 2000).

FIGURE 8-7: FRACTURES OF THE FEMUR

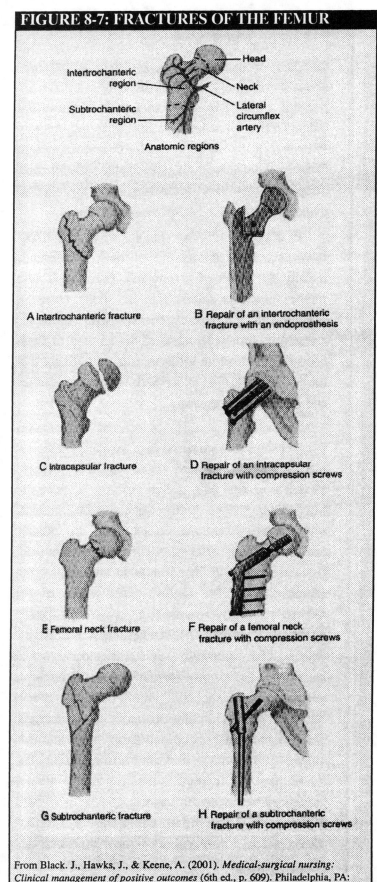

Anatomic regions

A Intertrochanteric fracture

B Repair of an intertrochanteric fracture with an endoprosthesis

C Intracapsular fracture

D Repair of an intracapsular fracture with compression screws

E Femoral neck fracture

F Repair of a femoral neck fracture with compression screws

G Subtrochanteric fracture

H Repair of a subtrochanteric fracture with compression screws

From Black. J., Hawks, J., & Keene, A. (2001). *Medical-surgical nursing: Clinical management of positive outcomes* (6th ed., p. 609). Philadelphia, PA: WB Saunders Co. Reprinted with permission from Elsevier.

The treatment of the fracture will be dependent upon several factors, including the type of fracture, the location, and whether it is an open or closed fracture. The patient's age and muscle size will also be determining factors. Because of the size of the femur and the strength of the thigh muscles, immobilizing the fracture and maintaining the alignment will require more than a cast.

Balanced suspension skeletal traction may be applied during the initial treatment period to reduce the fracture. The most common type of balanced suspension skeletal traction used for a fractured femur is the Thomas splint with Pearson attachment. If the traction is to be left in place until healing of the fracture occurs, it would need to remain intact for 8–12 weeks. Typically, however, after a few days of skeletal traction reduction, the patient undergoes an open reduction and internal fixation of the fracture, with the placement of intramedullary or interlocking nail devices. Internal fixation of the fracture is the preferred treatment of choice, as it allows for early ambulation and reduces the potential for complications (Ruda, 2000b). If the patient has experienced extensive soft tissue damage or bone loss, or multiple other traumas that do not allow the patient to undergo a surgical reduction and internal fixation, it may be necessary to apply an external fixation device to the femur instead.

If the fracture is located in the supracondylar area (distal third) of the femur, the fracture is likely to be treated initially with skeletal traction for 2–3 weeks until the pain and swelling is decreased. At that time, the traction is removed and the patient is fitted with a cast brace, which will provide immobilization and support of the fracture yet allow the patient earlier mobility with knee flexion and partial weight–bearing (Liddel, 2000b; Schoen, 2000).

Following successful reduction of the femoral fracture, two goals for all patients are to promote ambulation as early as possible and avoid complications. Following surgery for fixation of the fracture, the patient's leg will be placed in suspension traction for 2–3 days to provide support to the leg and promote comfort. While the patient is on bedrest, it is important for the nurse to position the patient in proper body alignment, observe for pressure points on the skin, and provide skin care at regular intervals. The patient should be assisted in altering position at least every 2 hours. Active and passive range of motion of all joints is performed as soon as allowed, and the patient is taught to do muscle setting exercises and ankle pumps hourly while awake. The patient is also encouraged to participate in the performance of activities of daily living within his or her limitations and to remain as independent in these activities as feasible. Upper extremity exercises are also important to help the patient develop muscle strength. Maintaining joint function and muscle strength will help the patient to ambulate using assistive devices such as crutches or walkers when walking can be resumed.

Tibia and Fibula

Tibia fractures can occur alone or in combination with the fracture of the fibula. Frequently in lower leg fractures, both bones are fractured together. It is uncommon for the fibula, which is a non-weight bearing bone, to be fractured alone. Due to the lack of protective muscle covering over the lower third of the tibia, it is common for fractures of the tibia to be open fractures. This portion of the tibia is also particularly susceptible to vascular damage, due to the lack of muscle (Schoen, 2000).

Fractures of the tibia and fibula are typically treated with either a closed reduction and a long leg cast; internal fixation and a long leg cast; or, in the case of soft tissue damage, external fixation (Schoen, 2000). The method of treatment will depend upon the type and location of fracture and the extent of tissue damage present.

Care of the patient following reduction is similar to care of the patient with a fractured femur. The affected extremity should be elevated to decrease swelling, and neurovascular checks are performed at a minimum of every 2 hours. Fractures of the tibia are especially prone to the development of compartment syndrome, so the nurse should closely assess the patient's affected extremity for increasing pain that is unrelieved by analgesics, increasing pain upon passive plantar flexion of the foot, paresthesia, pallor, decreased or absent pulses, and coolness of the extremity (Liddel, 2000b).

The patient will be allowed to begin ambulating with partial weight-bearing in about 7–10 days. After about 4–6 weeks, the long leg cast is removed, and a short leg cast is applied. This allows the patient to begin flexing and exercising the knee, thus decreasing knee stiffness. It takes about 10–12 weeks for the tibia to heal. If tissue and vascular damage is extensive, healing may be delayed, and the patient may require bone grafts to stimulate bone growth (Liddel, 2000b).

SUMMARY

While fractures can vary by location and type, there are several principles that are common to the nursing care of any patient who has experienced a fracture. Table 8–1 summarizes these principles. By incorporating these principles into the care of patients who have a fracture, nurses can ensure that patients are receiving quality care.

CASE STUDY

D.H. is a young male, age 22, who was involved in a motorcycle accident, resulting in the compound fracture of his left femur. He is hospitalized for treatment of the fractured femur, with his left leg being placed in skeletal traction using a Thomas splint and Pearson attachment to support the leg. Twenty-five pounds of weights have been applied to maintain the traction. He has been hospitalized for 2 days.

TABLE 8–1 PRINCIPLES OF NURSING CARE FOR PATIENTS WITH A FRACTURE

1. Decrease pain and promote comfort
2. Maintain satisfactory neurovascular status of affected body part
3. Decrease risk for infection
4. Maintain skin integrity
5. Maintain muscle strength and joint function
6. Encourage activity
7. Maintain adequate nutrition and fluid intake
8. Teach safety principles for use of assistive ambulatory devices (crutches, walkers)
9. Assess patient carefully for potential complications — fat emboli, pulmonary complications, infection, neurovascular compromise, compartment syndrome
10. Encourage independence and self-care as appropriate
11. Provide home care instructions to patient and significant others

Answer the following case study questions, writing your responses on a separate sheet of paper. Compare your responses to the answers that are located at the end of the chapter.

1. What nursing assessments would be appropriate for you to make on D.H. at this time?

2. Describe the advantages of treating D.H.'s fractured femur with skeletal traction.

3. You are observing D.H.'s position in bed and the alignment of the traction apparatus. What are the important points about his position and the alignment of the skeletal traction that you should be assessing?

4. What principles of nursing care should you incorporate into the plan of care for patients such as D.H. who have experienced a fracture?

5. You are providing pin care to the skeletal pin that is inserted in D.H.'s left femur for the traction. What assessments should you make about the pin and pin site while you are performing the pin care?

6. Describe the complications that D.H. can develop as a result of the skeletal traction.

7. In preparation for ambulation, what exercises should you encourage D.H. to perform?

Case Study Answers

1. The nursing assessments that are important at this stage of D.H's recovery include assessments that are specific to the fractured leg, as well as assessments related to D.H.'s potential for developing complications related to bedrest. A priority nursing assessment is the frequent evaluation of the neurovascular status of the fractured leg. The nurse should assess the neurovascular status of the leg at least every 4 hours and more frequently during the first 24 hours following the injury. A neurovascular assessment includes assessing the capillary filling time, temperature and color of the affected leg and foot, and palpating for peripheral pulses. Assessing for pain in the extremity, especially upon passive movement, sensation, and the ability to voluntarily move the foot are additional components of the neurovascular assessment. The nurse will also want to assess the patient for signs of infection due to the compound fracture and insertion of a skeletal pin. Because the patient is on bedrest, the nurse should assess the patient regularly for adverse effects related to bedrest. Lung sounds and bowel sounds should be assessed regularly. Fluid intake should be monitored and urinary output measured. The lower extremities should be assessed for indications of deep vein thrombosis. Skin should be inspected for areas of pressure development. The nurse should always assess the patient for fat embolism syndrome, which is most likely to develop within the first 24–48 hours following injury.

2. A major advantage of balanced suspension skeletal traction is that it provides direct pull on the fractured bone ends to achieve alignment.

Another advantage of skeletal traction is that it allows the patient more mobility in bed without disrupting the line of traction.

3. When assessing D.H.'s position in bed, the nurse should inspect the affected extremity to be sure that it is suspended off the bed and that the traction apparatus is not weighted down by bed linens. D.H. should be positioned in the center of the bed and in correct body alignment. Traction should be maintained without interruption. The traction weights should be hanging freely, and the counter traction should be maintained continuously. Ropes should move freely on the pulleys, and the rope knots should not be in contact with the pulleys.

4. Principles of care for the patient who has a fracture include:

   • decreasing pain and promoting comfort;

   • maintaining satisfactory neurovascular status of affected body part;

   • decreasing the risk for infection;

   • maintaining skin integrity;

   • maintaining muscle strength and joint function;

   • encouraging activity;

   • maintaining adequate nutrition and fluid intake;

   • teaching safety principles for use of assistive devices;

   • assessing for complications;

   • encouraging self-care as appropriate; and

   • providing home care instructions.

5. When providing skeletal pin care, the nurse must ensure that aseptic technique is used. The nurse should assess the insertion site for purulent drainage, redness, odor, or pain. There should not be any movement of the pin at the insertion site. If the nurse detects movement or sliding of the pin, this should be reported promptly to the physician. The nurse should assess the patient

for an elevated temperature, as this can be an indicator of an infection at the pin site, even before other, more obvious, signs of infection can be detected.

6. In addition to the complications that can result from bedrest, D.H. is susceptible to several complications as a result of having skeletal traction applied to a fractured femur. One potential complication of skeletal traction is nonunion of the bone fragments due to the application of too much traction, thus separating the bone fragments. Overriding of bone fragments can occur if not enough traction has been applied. Another potential complication is skin breakdown as a result of the patient's supine position in bed or of the traction apparatus applying pressure points at various locations on the affected extremity. The nurse should closely inspect the heel of the unaffected leg, the coccyx, and the elbows for skin breakdown due to the patient shifting position in bed. The traction apparatus can apply pressure to several different areas of the affected leg — the heel, Achilles tendon, popliteal area, lateral aspect of the knee, and the ischial tuberosity. The nurse should inspect these areas several times per shift to ensure that pressure areas are not developing. Additional complications include the potential for peroneal nerve damage, deep vein thrombosis, and infection.

7. The goal is to preserve muscle tone and strength as well as the function of the joints as much as possible. Passive and active range of motion should be performed each shift. Muscle setting exercises, such as gluteal setting and quadriceps setting, will help prepare the patient for ambulation as well as support circulation. Ankle circling or pumping exercises also support circulation. Upper extremity exercises will help D.H. prepare to support himself with a walker or crutches. An overhead trapeze attached to the bed frame will help D.H. maneuver himself in bed and maintain upper body strength.

EXAM QUESTIONS

CHAPTER 8
Questions 51-60

51. When providing discharge instructions to a patient who has fractured his clavicle, the nurse should tell the patient to

   a. exercise the fingers, wrist and elbow.

   b. do not lie supine until the clavicle has healed.

   c. perform shoulder shrugs every four hours.

   d. gently lift the affected arm over the head daily.

52. A patient with a distal humerus fracture that has been reduced and is newly casted is particularly susceptible to

   a. infection.

   b. compartment syndrome.

   c. fat emboli syndrome.

   d. malunion.

53. To encourage circulation and decrease swelling for a patient who has fractured his radius and has a long arm cast, the patient should

   a. apply ice to the affected extremity.

   b. perform pendulum exercises.

   c. sit in a high-Fowler's position.

   d. flex and extend fingers.

54. The nurse is caring for a patient on bedrest with a fractured pelvis. If the patient is allowed to turn, an appropriate way to accomplish this is to

   a. place the patient in a semi-sitting position by slightly raising the head of the bed.

   b. have the patient stand and bear weight.

   c. tilt the patient to the side at approximately 45 degrees and log roll.

   d. place the patient in the side lying SIMS position with the knee and thigh drawn upward.

55. To decrease pain from muscle spasms in a patient with a fractured spine, the nurse should

   a. apply heat to the area of the fracture.

   b. maintain the patient in a semi-Fowler's position.

   c. place an abductor pillow between the patient's legs.

   d. avoid frequent position changes.

56. The signs or symptoms of a possible fractured femur include

   a. excessive hip flexion.

   b. leg adduction.

   c. hyperextension of the knee.

   d. shortened length of extremity.

57. The most likely treatment to reduce the fractured femur of an adult patient initially is

    a. a long leg cast.

    b. suspension traction.

    c. balanced suspension skeletal traction.

    d. cast brace.

58. For a patient placed on bed rest to promote healing of a fractured femur, the nurse should

    a. encourage the patient's family to perform activities of daily living for the patient.

    b. teach the patient upper extremity exercises to maintain muscle strength.

    c. instruct the patient to do muscle setting exercises once a day.

    d. help the patient adjust position every 4 hours while awake.

59. A principle goal of nursing care for any patient who has a fracture is

    a. administer prophylactic antibiotics.

    b. maintain patient in supine position.

    c. promote patient self-care and independence.

    d. provide daily pin care.

60. A patient with a fractured tibia who complains of increased pain when the nurse places the patient's affected foot in a position of plantar flexion likely has

    a. a normal finding for a patient with a fractured tibia.

    b. a fracture that is not properly aligned.

    c. compartment syndrome.

    d. inadequate pain control.

CHAPTER 9

CARE OF PATIENTS WITH A FRACTURED HIP

CHAPTER OBJECTIVE

After completing this chapter, the reader will be able to describe the medical management and nursing care of patients who have experienced a fracture of the hip.

LEARNING OBJECTIVES

After studying this chapter, the reader will be able to

1. identify risk factors leading to the cause of a hip fracture.

2. specify the pathophysiology of a hip fracture.

3. identify the clinical manifestations of a hip fracture.

4. indicate the medical management of the patient who has experienced a fracture of the hip.

5. indicate the nursing care of the patient who has experienced a fracture of the hip.

6. identify the preoperative and postoperative care of the elderly patient who has experienced a hip fracture.

7. indicate the principles of rehabilitation for a patient who has experienced a fracture of the hip.

OVERVIEW

Hip fractures are a common medical problem in the elderly population and a significant cause of mortality and morbidity among the elderly in the United States. For many elderly people, suffering a hip fracture has come to symbolize the onset of disability, loss of independence, and the end of a productive life. It is estimated that hip fractures annually cost the United States 7–10 billion dollars (Roberts, 2001). Many of those who suffer a hip fracture are women who have osteoporosis. Many individuals also have a co-existing health problem — for example, cardiovascular disease, chronic respiratory problems, diabetes — which complicates recovery from the fracture. The potential for full functional recovery is dependent upon the patient's condition prior to the injury and the avoidance of complications postoperatively. Nurses have a significant role in preparing the patient prior to surgery and supporting postoperative recovery. This chapter discusses the nursing care for a patient who has experienced a hip fracture.

ETIOLOGY OF HIP FRACTURES

The majority of hip fractures, over 90%, are associated with a fall (Roberts, 2001). Women who have developed low density bone mass due to osteoporosis are particularly susceptible to fracturing a hip and falling. Many falls are caused by hazards in the environment, such as throw rugs, poor lighting, uneven walking surfaces, and slippery floors. Some elderly people may also have difficulty seeing or may take medications that predispose them to unsteady gaits or lightheadedness.

As a means of preventing falls and decreasing the potential for a fracture, it is important that individuals and their families understand how to make a living environment safer for an elderly person — eliminating uneven, slippery surfaces, removing loose rugs, installing safety equipment in bathrooms, ensuring good lighting, and using good-fitting shoes. If the individual uses assistive devices to ambulate, these devices should be in good repair and used correctly. These initiatives help decrease the potential for a fall to occur in the home environment.

PATHOPHYSIOLOGY

Fractures of the hip are classified into two categories: 1) intracapsular fractures, which occur within the joint capsule in the neck of the femur and 2) extracapsular fractures, which occur outside the joint capsule. These fractures can be further subdivided within their categories. Intracapsular fractures can be subcapital, transcervical, or basilar neck fractures, depending upon which region of the femoral neck is fractured. Extracapsular fractures are classified as intertrochanteric (occurring between the greater and lesser trochanters) and subtrochanteric (occurring below the lesser trochanter). The intracapsular fractures are more likely to be associated with less traumatic events and osteoporosis, and they are more common in the frail elderly. Extracapsular fractures are more likely to be caused by significant traumatic events resulting in a direct blow such as a fall (Ruda, 2000b). Figure 9–1 illustrates these various fracture sites in the hip.

The location of the fracture can make a difference in the healing process. Intracapsular fractures, for example, can lead to an interruption of the blood supply to the femoral head and cause avascular necrosis, delayed union or nonunion of the bone. The extracapsular region has a much richer blood supply, so fractures that occur in the intertrochan-

teric area are likely to heal rapidly (Liddel, 2000b). However, because intertrochanteric fractures are more likely to be caused by a serious traumatic event, there is more likelihood that the fracture itself will be comminuted (Liddel, 2000b) and develop the complication of malunion, resulting in a shortened extremity (Marek, 1999).

The overwhelming majority of hip fractures occur in either the intertrochanteric or femoral neck area. Only about 10% of all hip fractures occur in the subtrochanteric region (Marek, 1999b).

CLINICAL MANIFESTATIONS OF A HIP FRACTURE

The clinical manifestations of a hip fracture include external rotation of the hip and a shortened extremity. The patient is unable to bear weight on the leg and will usually complain of severe pain and tenderness in the area of the fracture (Roberts, 2001). A hematoma or ecchymosis may develop (Liddel, 2000b). Depending upon the cause of the fracture, there could be soft tissue trauma present as well. The presence of a fracture will be confirmed by an x-ray.

MEDICAL MANAGEMENT OF A HIP FRACTURE

Upon confirmation of the hip fracture, the treatment of choice is surgical intervention, unless the patient's condition contraindicates surgery. Surgical treatment helps to ensure proper reduction and alignment of the bone ends, mobilizes the patient more quickly, and decreases the likelihood that the patient will develop complications. Patients with a hip fracture who are treated by traction alone require 8–12 weeks, or more, for healing to occur, and they are especially prone to the hazards of immobility. Patients who are treated surgically are usually transferred from the bed to a chair on the

FIGURE 9-1: FRACTURES OF THE HIP

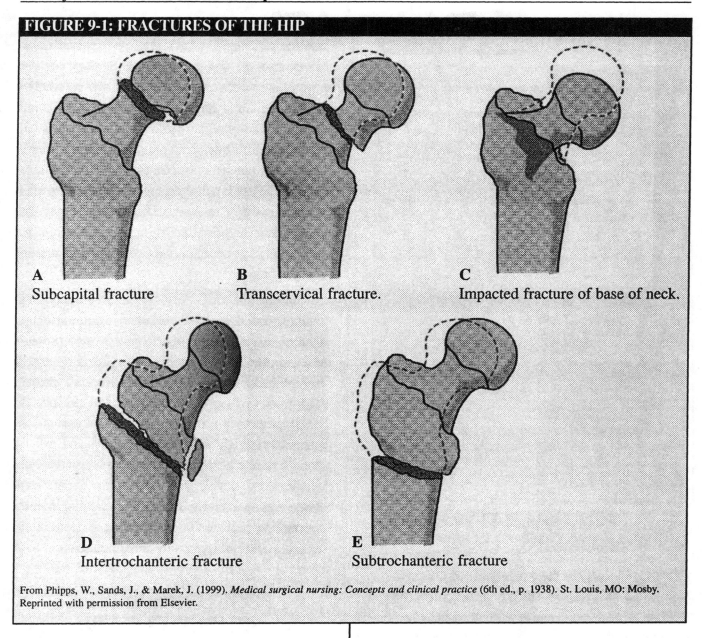

A
Subcapital fracture

B
Transcervical fracture.

C
Impacted fracture of base of neck.

D
Intertrochanteric fracture

E
Subtrochanteric fracture

From Phipps, W., Sands, J., & Marek, J. (1999). *Medical surgical nursing: Concepts and clinical practice* (6th ed., p. 1938). St. Louis, MO: Mosby. Reprinted with permission from Elsevier.

first postoperative day, which helps minimize the complications resulting from immobility.

There are several surgical procedures that may be used, depending upon the location and type of fracture (see Figure 9–2). Intracapsular fractures are usually surgically treated with the insertion of a femoral head prosthesis. The femoral head is removed, and a prosthetic femoral head is inserted in its place. By removing the femoral head and replacing it with a prosthesis, the surgeon can avoid the complications of avascular necrosis and nonunion (Liddel, 2000b). Extracapsular fractures are more likely to be pinned, using pins, screws and plates, or nails to accomplish the pinning. This procedure is called an ORIF, for open reduction and internal fixation (Ruda, 2000b). Whichever surgical procedure is used, the best time period for performing the surgery is within 12–24 hours of the injury, as long as the patient is in a favorable condition for surgery. Prior to surgery, the fracture may be temporarily immobilized by the use of Buck's traction.

FIGURE 9-2: TYPES OF INTERNAL FIXATION FOR A HIP FRACTURE.

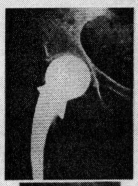

A
Femoral head endoprosthesis.

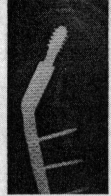

B
Type of hip compression screw with side plate

From Lewis, S., Heitkemper, M., & Dirksen, S. (2000). *Medical-surgical nursing: Assessment and management of clinical problems* (5th ed., p. 1789). St. Louis, MO: Mosby. Reprinted with permission from Elsevier.

PREOPERATIVE NURSING CARE

Prior to surgery for a fractured hip, the patient must be assessed for the presence of chronic health problems that can negatively impact the postoperative recovery. Elderly patients are especially likely to have co-existing health conditions such as coronary artery disease, hypertension, diabetes, and chronic obstructive pulmonary disease. The physician will evaluate the health status of the patient and stabilize any known medical problems prior to taking the patient to surgery.

Both the patient and family members need education about what to expect before, during, and after surgery. The patient will need to know what will be expected postoperatively regarding mobility. The importance of maintaining the range of motion and the muscle strength of all unaffected extremities

should be emphasized. The nurse can demonstrate how the patient will be asked to move in bed, transfer techniques, and any assistive devices, such as trapeze overheads and walkers, that will be used by the patient. The patient also needs to know about any position or weight-bearing restrictions that will be required following surgery. The nurse should emphasize that pain medication will be available and administered to the patient to help decrease pain when moving. The nurse should also begin discharge planning prior to surgery, so that the patient and family can anticipate what to expect during the recovery phase.

During the time period prior to surgery, pain medication and muscle relaxants are administered to decrease pain and muscle spasms and promote the comfort of the patient. The fractured hip is immobilized, usually by temporary Buck's traction. The nurse will provide skin care to prevent the development of pressure ulcers, encourage the patient to cough and breathe deeply, and ask the patient to use incentive spirometry to decrease the chances of developing hypostatic pneumonia. Encouraging exercise to maintain circulation in the extremities will also be appropriate to decrease the chances of developing a thromboembolism.

POSTOPERATIVE NURSING CARE

Postoperatively, the nursing care of the patient will be similar to any patient who has undergone surgery, focusing on the prevention of postoperative complications. The nurse will monitor vital signs carefully, encourage coughing and deep breathing every 1–2 hours, monitor intravenous fluids as well as intake and output, administer pain medication, and assess the wound dressing for bleeding (Ruda, 2000b). Prophylactic intravenous antibiotics may be prescribed to decrease the potential for infection. Abduction splints or pillows should be placed between the legs to help maintain the hips in a position of abduction and promote alignment of the hip. The hip is also maintained in a position of neutral rotation. Pneumatic compression devices applied to the lower extremities will help prevent venous pooling and clot formation (Liddel, 2000b). Prophylactic anticoagulant therapy may also be prescribed to decrease the likelihood of clot formation.

The nurse must monitor carefully the patient for signs of neurovascular impairment during the immediate postoperative phase. Neurovascular impairment can develop due to trauma to blood vessels or nerves, either from the traumatic injury or the surgery. Assessing the peripheral pulses, skin color, temperature, capillary refill, sensation, and movement of the affected extremity at frequent intervals and comparing findings to the unaffected extremity is an essential nursing responsibility.

Pain management in the immediate postoperative period and beyond is another important nursing task. Uncontrolled pain can impact the patient's ability to move in bed or be mobile, leading to the development of postoperative complications. Postoperative acute pain management in the elderly patient is sometimes overlooked. This may be due to the fact that the elderly are less likely to report pain, may express pain in ways that are different from the general population, and may be cognitively impaired and unable to verbalize the need for pain medication (MacDonald & Hilton, 2001). It is important that all nursing staff be alert to the potential indicators that the patient is experiencing pain or discomfort, whether or not this patient can verbalize it. Nonverbal indications can be highly individual, but they are likely to include restlessness, agitation, and a reluctance to move. Analgesics should be administered as needed, and the patient's response to the medication should be carefully evaluated and documented. If the prescribed analgesic produces inadequate pain control, this should be promptly reported to the physician so that more effective pain management can be achieved. Moving the affected extremity gently and providing adequate support to

the extremity while maintaining alignment will also help promote patient comfort.

The most common complication occurring after surgery for a hip fracture is the development of a deep vein thrombosis (DVT). The nurse should be aggressive in encouraging fluid intake to 2500mL/day or more, to decrease the potential for dehydration and hemoconcentration. Foot pedaling and ankle circling exercises should be performed hourly; the patient will need to be reminded of the importance of performing these exercises. Family members can also be instructed to remind the patient to exercise. The sequential decompressing devices should be used as ordered; antiembolism hose may also be applied. The nurse must ensure that the equipment is functioning properly and that the antiembolism hose are wrinkle-free. The patient's legs should be assessed for DVT every 4 hours, and any signs of redness, tenderness, swelling, or low-grade temperature should be promptly reported. Anticoagulant therapy may also be prescribed as a prophylactic measure (Ruda, 2000b).

Another potential complication following hip surgery is the onset of respiratory problems, especially the development of pneumonia. The nurse should auscultate breath sounds every 4–8 hours to detect any adventitious breath sounds and, as indicated previously, encourage frequent coughing and deep breathing. The patient should also be assisted with using incentive spirometry every hour while awake. Changing the patient's position every 2 hours is another appropriate nursing intervention.

Frequent change of positions will also help decrease the potential for the development of pressure ulcers. The patient will not be able to change positions independently following surgery; he or she will need the assistance of nursing personnel. It is important that the patient not be allowed to lie in any one position for longer than 2 hours. The nurse should closely inspect the patient's skin after turning, noting any prolonged redness that does not resolve itself within 15 minutes after the repositioning. If the redness is not resolved within the 15 minutes after turning, it indicates that the patient must be turned more frequently. A turning schedule should be established that is individualized to the patient's needs, and this schedule should be clearly communicated to all shifts.

Areas particularly susceptible to skin breakdown following hip fracture surgery, which require careful monitoring and skin care, include the coccyx, scapulae, elbows, and heels, but any bony prominence has the potential for breakdown. The skin should be kept clean and dry. When turning and repositioning the patient, care should be taken not to create friction on the skin, instead, efforts should be made to decrease shearing forces. Even if specialty beds or other protective devices such as heel protectors are used for the patient, the importance of maintaining a turning schedule and visually inspecting the patient's skin at each turning and repositioning does not diminish.

The onset of confusion, or delirium, is another potential patient complication following hip surgery. This is a relatively common and serious problem, as it can contribute to a prolonged recovery period and lead to functional decline in the patient. The onset of this delirium is most likely to develop within the first 5 postoperative days (Milisen et al., 2002). Many patients who experience delirium following surgery have never before experienced any confusion. The etiology is unclear, but delirium could stem from a different environment, decreased oxygenation, sensory overload or deprivation, medications, pain, and a disruption in the patient's regular routine (Roberts, 2001).

Initial indications of the onset of delirium may include forgetfulness, lack of attention, fear, or disorientation. It is important for the nurse to assess the patient carefully for the onset of these behaviors and to implement actions that will help maintain the patient's orientation to the environment. Using clocks and calendars will help the patient keep track of time. Ensuring that the patient has access to hear-

ing aids and glasses will help keep the patient in touch with the environment. It is also helpful to establish a day-night routine for the patient, scheduling minimal disruptions during the nighttime so that the patient can re-establish a more normal wake-sleep cycle. All medications that the patient receives should be monitored for their potential to cause confusion.

Complications that can occur later in the recovery phase following surgery, especially with a femoral neck fracture, include avascular necrosis and nonunion of the fracture. Infection, dislocation of the prosthetic head, and loosening of internal fixation hardware are other potential complications.

REHABILITATION FOLLOWING HIP SURGERY

Rehabilitation following hip surgery for a fracture is very individualized to the patient. The patient will likely remain hospitalized for about 4 days following the surgery. Most patients will be discharged from the hospital to a long-term care facility as they continue their recovery. How quickly the patient will be able to regain function depends on several factors. Some of the factors affecting recovery include the patient's age, health status prior to the injury and surgery, mental status, presence of depression, and the type of fracture. Patients who experience cognitive impairment are more likely to have a poorer outcome following surgery and face the potential for placement in a long-term care facility with decreased function and increased mortality (Feldt & Finch, 2002).

It is important to the patient's long-term recovery that mobility begin early in the postoperative period. Physical therapy will be key to the patient being able to ambulate safely. The nurse is responsible for reinforcing what the patient is taught by the physical therapist. Emphasis will be placed on maintaining the range of motion, muscle strength, and tone of the muscles in the unaffected extremities. The patient will be encouraged to use the overhead trapeze on the bed as much as possible to strengthen the arms, as the patient is going to need upper body strength to safely use any assistive walking devices. Gluteal setting exercises and quadriceps setting exercises will also be taught. Adequate muscle strength throughout the body will be key to successful ambulation following surgery.

Ambulation will usually be started the first or second postoperative day. On the first postoperative day, the patient will be helped out of bed and placed in a chair. Following success with sitting in the chair, the patient will begin to ambulate with assistance. The amount of weight that the patient will be allowed to place on the affected leg will be stipulated by the surgeon's order and depends upon the stability of the reduction and procedure performed. However, the nurse can anticipate that the patient will be restricted to non-weight bearing or only partial weight-bearing early in the recovery phase. The amount of weight-bearing that the leg will be allowed to tolerate will gradually increase to full

weight-bearing as healing progresses. The patient will require the use of crutches or a walker when ambulating.

The physical therapist will teach the patient how to transfer out of bed safely and how to use the crutches or walker to ambulate. Many patients will use a walker, as they require more stability and support than crutches will provide. Table 9–1 identifies safety principles related to ambulating with a walker. The patient will require a great deal of encouragement to persevere in learning to ambulate following the surgery. Pain, anxiety, fatigue, and lack of strength can be difficult to overcome without the encouragement of health care providers and family members.

If the patient has had the femoral head replaced with a prosthetic device, there will be certain precautions to be followed to prevent the dislocation of the device. Some precautions will also apply to patients who have had a hip pinning, but the fear of dislocation does not exist with these patients. When turning the patient in bed or getting the patient up to ambulate, care should be taken that the affected hip is not adducted. The leg should always be main-

TABLE 9–1: SAFETY PRINCIPLES FOR AMBULATING WITH A WALKER

- Encourage patient to regularly perform upper extremity strengthening exercises.
- Patient should wear comfortable, low heel, firm walking shoes.
- Use a gait belt if there is concern about the patient's balance and stability.
- The height of the walker should be slightly below waist height and allow for slight flexion in elbow.
- When rising from sitting position, the patient should push off from bed or chair and then place hands on walker one at a time. Do not use walker to pull up from sitting position as it is unstable.
- Advance walker and affected extremity at the same time, using arms to support weight as needed. Then advance unaffected extremity to walker.
- Caution patient not to advance walker too far ahead of the unaffected extremity; avoid leaning forward into walker.
- Do not advance unaffected extremity until all points of the walker are securely on the ground.
- Periodically inspect walker tips and walker bolts and screws for wear and looseness.
- To sit in a chair, turn around and back up to the chair until the unaffected extremity touches the chair. Then reach for chair arms to lower self into chair — do not use walker for support while sitting down as it is unstable.
- Nurses or assistants should assist patient with ambulation by standing to the side and slightly behind the patient.

tained in a position of neutral rotation as well. The patient should also be careful not to flex the hip past 90 degrees, as this can place strain on any pinning devices and can predispose the patient to dislocation of the prosthetic device, if one was used. The patient should be cautioned against sitting in any soft, low chairs, as these will place the hip in a flexed position greater than 90 degrees.

Table 9–2 describes the precautions that a patient who has had a femoral-head prosthesis inserted should follow postoperatively.

TABLE 9-2: FEMORAL-HEAD PROSTHESIS

Do Not
- Force hip into greater than 90 degrees of flexion*
- Force hip into adduction
- Force hip into internal rotation
- Cross legs
- Put on own shoes or stockings until 8 wk after surgery without adaptive device (e.g., long-handled shoehorn or stocking-helper)
- Sit on chairs without arms to aid rising to a standing position*

Do
- Use toilet elevator on toilet seat•
- Place chair inside shower or tub and remain seated while washing
- Use pillow between legs for first 8 wk after surgery when lying on "good" side or when supine*
- Keep hip in neutral, straight position when sitting, walking, or lying*
- Notify surgeon if severe pain, deformity, or loss of function occurs*
- Inform dentist of presence of prosthesis before dental work so that prophylactic antibiotics can be given

* These precautions may also apply after a hip pinning.

From Lewis, S., Heitkemper, M., & Dirksen, S. (2000). *Medical-surgical nursing: Assessment and management of clinical problems* (5th ed., p. 1793). St. Louis, MO: Mosby. Reprinted with permission from Elsevier.

As elderly patients are transferred to long-term care facilities to continue their recovery from a hip fracture, it is important to remember that the patients still need adequate pain control. Studies have indicated that patients do not receive as much analgesia as they require to control pain when they rehabilitate following surgery. The increased expectations for ambulation and activity will lead to an increase in discomfort (Feldt & Gunderson, 2002). It is important that the nursing staff understands this need for continued and increased pain control and that they ensure their patients receive the appropriate analgesics. It is also important that the patients and their families understand the importance of requesting pain medication. The nurse has a responsibility to serve as a patient advocate to ensure that the patient receives the appropriate standard of care. The care plans of all patients must include a plan for adequate pain control throughout the acute and rehabilitation phases of the patient's recovery.

It is also important that the nurse help the patient adjust to the restrictions in activity and the loss of independence that the patient is experiencing. For some patients, a hip fracture may mean that they will not be able to return to independent living in their own home. It is common for patients to experience depression or to feel that they have lost control over the situation in which they find themselves. The nurse can provide information on community resources the patient and family can use to get discharge planning assistance with any concerns related to rehabilitation or post-rehabilitation care. Many patients have concerns about finances or how to make environmental safety modifications to their living environment. In-home health care assistance or assistance with the activities of daily living, such as care of the home, grocery shopping, or transportation, may also be a concern. It is essential that the nurse provide the patient with the opportunity to express such concerns. Social services, support groups, and clergy are all potential resources for the patient and family. Allaying the patient's concerns about these types of issues can have a positive outcome on the extent of the patient's recovery.

SUMMARY

A hip fracture is a life-altering event for many elderly patients. This chapter discussed the etiology and pathophysiology of hip fractures as well as the medical management and nursing care appropriate for patients who have experienced a hip fracture. The quality of the nursing care received by the patient following hip surgery for a fracture will, in many cases, be a determining factor in the patient's ultimate outcome for recovery. The nurse is responsible for developing and implementing a plan of care to prevent the many postoperative complications that can develop for a patient who has a hip fracture. On-going nursing assessment and monitoring of the patient's condition is essential to ensure a recovery with fewer complications.

CASE STUDY

Mrs. F.C. is a 78 year-old female who has been admitted to the hospital with a suspected fracture of the left hip. Upon assessment of the left leg, you observe that the left leg is shorter than the right leg, and the left leg also appears to be externally rotated. She is complaining of severe left hip pain. Her B/P is 134/72, pulse 74 and respirations 16. She is afebrile. Both feet are warm to touch and bilateral pedal pulses are easily palpated, 2+ in strength. A hip x-ray confirms a left hip intracapsular fracture in the subcapital region of the femoral neck. Mrs. F.C. is scheduled to have a femoral head prosthesis inserted to repair the left hip.

Answer the following case study questions, writing your responses on a separate sheet of paper. Compare your responses to the answers that are located at the end of the chapter.

1. What are the risk factors associated with a hip fracture?

2. Prior to surgery, what preoperative nursing care would be appropriate for Mrs. F.C.?

3. Buck's traction has been applied to Mrs. F. C.'s left leg. What nursing care should you implement for Mrs. F. C. while she is in traction?

4. Mrs. F.C. has a femoral head prosthesis inserted to repair her left hip. How does this surgery differ from an open reduction and internal fixation procedure, which is also used to treat hip fractures?

5. What position should Mrs. F. C.'s left leg be maintained in following surgery?

6. What are common postoperative complications for patients who have had hip surgery?

7. What patient care instructions should the nurse give Mrs. F. C. to avoid dislocation of the hip prosthesis?

Answers to Case Study

1. Hip fractures are a common health problem for the elderly in the U.S. The majority of these hip fractures are associated with a fall. Women with osteoporosis are particularly vulnerable to hip fractures.

2. Preoperative nursing care will include assessing Mrs. F.C. for the presence of other chronic health problems, which may negatively impact her recovery from surgery, and stabilizing these conditions. A major preoperative nursing goal will be to decrease pain and promote comfort. The nurse will administer analgesics and muscle relaxants to decrease pain and relieve muscle spasms. The nurse will also immobilize the hip to minimize discomfort. Buck's traction may be applied temporarily to immobilize the hip. While awaiting surgery, the nurse should provide skin care to prevent skin breakdown; encourage coughing, deep breathing, and incentive spirometry to prevent hypostatic pneumonia; and encourage exercises, such as ankle circling, to promote circulation. In addition, the nurse should also teach the patient and family members about what to expect postoperatively, especially regarding mobility and positioning.

3. Nursing care for a patient with Buck's traction includes ensuring that the traction is not applied so tightly that it impairs the circulation. Neurovascular checks should be performed frequently, at least every 2 hours. The patient will be maintained in a supine position. As a result, the patient in Buck's traction is prone to skin breakdown, and the nurse must carefully inspect bony prominences and provide skin care at least every 2 hours. Once every shift, the Buck's traction should be carefully removed for the nurse to provide skin care. Manual traction is applied until Buck's traction is reapplied. The nurse should also ensure that the traction weights hang freely and do not touch the floor.

4. Intracapsular fractures are usually treated by removal of the femoral head and insertion of a femoral head prosthesis. With the removal of the femoral head and insertion of a prosthesis, the surgeon can avoid the potential complications of avascular necrosis and nonunion of the bone fragments. Extracapsular fractures are more likely to be repaired by an open reduction and internal fixation, which requires the insertion of pins, screws and plates, or nails to stabilize the fracture.

5. Following surgery, Mrs. F.C.'s left hip should be maintained in a position of abduction and neutral rotation. Abduction splints or pillows can be used to help the patient maintain this position.

6. The most common postoperative complications following hip surgery is deep vein thrombosis, followed by pneumonia, pressure ulcers, and confusion.

7. To avoid dislocation of the femoral prosthesis, Mrs. F.C. should be instructed not to cross the leg over the midline of the body (adduction) and not to flex the hip past 90 degrees. She should avoid low seats and soft chairs.

EXAM QUESTIONS

CHAPTER 9
Questions 61-66

61. One risk factor for a hip fracture is

    a. lack of activity.

    b. hypercalcemia.

    c. osteoarthritis.

    d. osteoporosis.

62. A fractured hip may be indicated by

    a. one leg that is longer than the other.

    b. the hip being externally rotated.

    c. the leg being in adduction.

    d. the hip being flexed.

63. The treatment of choice for a patient who has experienced an extracapsular hip fracture is

    a. surgical pinning.

    b. insertion of a prosthetic femoral head.

    c. skeletal traction.

    d. total hip replacement.

64. Prior to surgery for a hip fracture, the nurse will anticipate the patient being placed in

    a. skeletal traction.

    b. a long leg cast.

    c. Buck's traction.

    d. pelvic traction.

65. After surgery for a fractured hip, the nurse will carefully position the patient so that the affected hip stays in

    a. external rotation.

    b. internal rotation.

    c. adduction.

    d. abduction.

66. Slower rehabilitation from hip surgery is most likely to result from a situation where

    a. the surgery to repair the hip was delayed for 24 hours following the injury.

    b. the patient develops cognitive impairment following surgery.

    c. the surgeon inserts screws and plates into the hip instead of a prosthetic device.

    d. the patient cannot ambulate without the use of a walker.

CHAPTER 10

CARE OF PATIENTS WITH OSTEOMYELITIS

CHAPTER OBJECTIVE

After completing this chapter, the reader will be able to describe the medical management and nursing care of patients who have osteomyelitis. In addition, the prevention of osteomyelitis is addressed.

LEARNING OBJECTIVES

After studying this chapter, the reader will be able to

1. identify the risk factors for the development of osteomyelitis.

2. define the etiology and pathophysiology of osteomyelitis.

3. specify the clinical manifestations of osteomyelitis.

4. select the medical management and nursing care of patients with osteomyelitis.

5. indicate preventive steps that can be taken to prevent the development of osteomyelitis.

OVERVIEW

Osteomyelitis is an infection of the bone. Osteomyelitis can be very serious and difficult to treat, leading to chronic disease and disability. In the United States, the majority of osteomyelitis cases are caused by direct penetration (Schoen,

2000). This chapter focuses on the medical management and nursing care of patients who have developed acute osteomyelitis. The prevention of osteomyelitis is also addressed.

ETIOLOGY

Bacteria are the most common cause of osteomyelitis, especially *Staphylococcus aureus*. However, other bacteria such as *Pseudomonas*, *Klebsiella*, *Salmonella*, and *Escherichia coli* can be causative agents (Roberts & Lappe, 2000). Viruses, fungi, and parasites can also lead to the development of osteomyelitis (Marek, 1999b).

Bone has several structural factors that make it difficult to treat osteomyelitis. The microscopic channels present in the bone do not allow access by the body's natural defense cells, thus allowing organisms to readily proliferate. The bone's microcirculation is easily damaged and destroyed by bacterial toxins. This impairs blood flow in the bone and leads to bone ischemia and necrosis. And finally, it is difficult for new bone to be formed to replace necrotic bone tissue and the integrity of the bone structure is weakened (McCance & Mourad, 2000b). Because it is difficult to treat osteomyelitis, prevention of osteomyelitis in the first place is the best treatment.

Osteomyelitis results from organisms that enter bone tissue from either exogenous sources or endogenous sources. Exogenous sources are from outside the body. Infections from exogenous sources can come from open fractures, surgery (especially total joint replacements), or puncture wounds. Animal or human bites can also introduce bacteria to the body that spreads to the bone. People with chronic health conditions such as drug/alcohol abuse, diabetes, or immunosuppression are more susceptible to developing osteomyelitis (Marek, 1999b). Those who are poorly nourished are also more susceptible to osteomyelitis (Liddel, 2000b).

Endogenous sources of osteomyelitis, also known as hematogenous osteomyelitis, originate within the body and are blood-borne. Common sources of infection within the body are oral, respiratory, ear, sinus, gastrointestinal, and genitourinary (Marek, 1999b). Children and the elderly are more susceptible to this form of osteomyelitis.

Whatever the etiology, it is important for the nurse to remember that osteomyelitis is very difficult to treat, especially if it is undetected in the early stages. Nurses should be particularly vigilant in assessing for osteomyelitis in all patients who are considered to be at risk. If osteomyelitis is not treated promptly in its acute stage, it can progress to chronic osteomyelitis and lead to loss of function, amputation, and even death.

PATHOPHYSIOLOGY

In osteomyelitis, the infectious organism invades the bone tissue and initiates an inflammatory response. The inflammatory response leads to the development of edema and increased vascularity in the area. Leukocytes migrate to the site, and inflammatory exudate collects at the site and forms an abscess. Due to the vascular engorgement that develops, the vessels in the area thrombose and the blood flow to the site is compromised. As the site of infection expands and the exudate continues to grow, pressure develops at the site, leading to ischemia of the bone and eventually necrosis. The exudate extends into the medullary cavity and under the periosteum, stripping the periosteum off the bone

and further compromising the vascular supply of underlying bone tissue. This complication is more likely to occur in children. Bacteria can also escape from the dead bone tissue into the surrounding soft tissue and invade nearby joints (McCance & Mourad, 2000).

The necrotic bone that develops forms an area referred to as *sequestrum*. The sequestrum is separated from the surrounding bone that is still living; it provides an area for bacteria to continue to live. With the continued existence of bacteria in the sequestrum, chronic osteomyelitis develops.

In response to bone destruction and disruption of the periosteum, the body initiates an intense osteoblastic activity. The osteoblasts stimulate the growth of new bone, which surrounds and encloses the area of dead bone. The new bone which surrounds the sequestrum is referred to as *involucrum* (McCance & Mourad, 2000). In effect, the sequestrum, with its infected bone, is now walled-off and difficult to reach with blood-borne leukocytes or antibiotic therapy. Sinus tracts can develop, however, allowing bacterial exudate to escape from the sequestrum and invade surrounding tissues. The sequestrum can remain present in the bone as chronic osteomyelitis, periodically leading to abscess formation throughout the remainder of the patient's life. Figure 10–1 depicts the development of osteomyelitis with the presence of sequestrum and involucrum.

CLINICAL MANIFESTATIONS OF OSTEOMYELITIS

Acute Osteomyelitis

The onset of acute osteomyelitis can be sudden. The patient will likely exhibit both local and systemic manifestations of the infection. Locally the involved area will be swollen, tender, and warm to touch. The patient will experience severe pain, espe-

FIGURE 10-1: DEVELOPMENT OF OSTEOMYELITIS INFECTION WITH INVOLUCRUM AND SEQUESTRUM

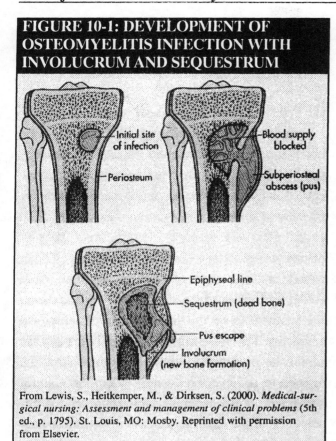

From Lewis, S., Heitkemper, M., & Dirksen, S. (2000). *Medical-surgical nursing: Assessment and management of clinical problems* (5th ed., p. 1795). St. Louis, MO: Mosby. Reprinted with permission from Elsevier.

cially upon movement. Systemic manifestations include fever, chills, and a feeling of malaise, which are indications of septicemia. The patient may also experience night sweats and nausea (Ruda, 2000b).

Chronic Osteomyelitis

Acute osteomyelitis that lasts longer than 1 month is categorized as chronic osteomyelitis (Ruda, 2000b). Chronic osteomyelitis develops when the bone infection has not been effectively treated in the acute stage. Manifestations of chronic osteomyelitis can recur at intermittent intervals. When symptoms are active, the patient will complain of pain, swelling, and other signs of inflammation. The area may also have a draining sinus wound (Liddel, 2000b). Chronic osteomyelitis is difficult to treat, as the area of chronic infection is not accessible to antibiotic therapy.

DIAGNOSIS OF OSTEOMYELITIS

Diagnosis of osteomyelitis is made through laboratory studies, cultures, and x-rays. The patient will exhibit an elevated leukocyte count and sedimentation rate. Wound cultures and blood cultures will also be conducted to identify the causative organism and to determine the organism's sensitivity to antibiotic therapy (Liddel, 2000b). Standard x-rays will not reveal evidence of osteomyelitis until at least 10–14 days after the onset of the infection. Delaying a diagnosis of osteomyelitis will adversely affect the success of treatment. Bone scans, however, can detect the presence of osteomyelitis approximately 24–72 hours after the onset. MRIs can also detect osteomyelitis at an earlier stage (Ruda, 2000b).

MEDICAL MANAGEMENT

The goal of medical management of osteomyelitis is to treat the infection as early as possible and eradicate the organism. Prompt identification of an antibiotic that the organism will be sensitive to is essential. It is important to begin antibiotic therapy prior to the onset of bone ischemia and necrosis. Once the blood supply to the bone is compromised, the antibiotic will not be able to reach the area of infection via the bloodstream. The antibiotics will be aggressively administered intravenously for approximately 6 weeks. Following intravenous administration, the antibiotics will be given orally for up to an additional 6 months of therapy (Liddel, 2000b).

If antibiotic therapy alone is not effective, the necrotic bone area may need to be surgically excised. Following removal of the infected bone tissue, a closed wound irrigation system may be inserted to provide continuous wound irrigation with antibiotics and promote the further removal of tissue debris. If the osteomyelitis has occurred as a result of the insertion of a total joint prosthesis, the prosthesis may need to be removed to adequately treat the infection (Ruda, 2000b).

If the surgically debrided area is large, the wound may need to be temporarily packed with antibiotic-impregnated beads to treat the infection (Ruda, 2000b). After the infection is eradicated, bone and/or skin grafts may be necessary to promote healing of the wound. This surgical reconstruction of the wound may take place in several stages over a period of time. Hyperbaric oxygen therapy may also be used to treat chronic osteomyelitis.

In addition to treatment to eradicate the infection, the patient will need analgesics for the severe pain. The affected extremity is also immobilized to promote comfort and decrease the likelihood of further injury to the bone. Bone that is infected is weak and at high risk for developing pathological fractures (Ruda, 2000b). External fixation devices may be used to stabilize the affected bone.

NURSING CARE OF THE PATIENT WITH OSTEOMYELITIS

A patient who has osteomyelitis is seriously ill and usually experiencing much discomfort. A priority goal of nursing care is to relieve the patient's pain and promote comfort. The nurse should make sure that the patient understands the need to take analgesics to control the pain. Analgesics must be administered prior to the pain level becoming severe. Other measures that can help decrease the pain are immobilizing the affected part and ensuring adequate support through the use of splints. Warm compresses may also be used to promote comfort. When moving the affected part, the nurse should always be sure to support the body part both above and below the area of infection. This provides stability and support of the body part and decreases stress on the bone. It also decreases the likelihood of a pathologi-

cal fracture. Keeping the body part elevated whenever possible and maintaining proper alignment will also decrease pain. The patient is likely to be on bedrest during the acute phase of illness if the infection is in a lower extremity.

Another priority nursing goal is to monitor the patient's response to the antibiotic therapy and support wound healing. It is essential that the intravenous antibiotics be administered promptly to maintain a constant therapeutic blood level. All wound care and dressing changes must be performed using sterile asepsis to prevent further wound contamination. A patient with an open wound and exposed bone is highly compromised and susceptible to the introduction of additional organisms. The nurse must understand the rationale behind the prescribed wound care and follow the regimen to achieve the desired outcomes. Careful assessment of the wound's appearance and documentation of the findings are also important to help evaluate the effectiveness of the prescribed therapy. Proper nutrition with a diet high in vitamin C and protein, as well as adequate fluid intake, will be necessary to support wound healing.

While the patient is immobilized, it is important to maintain functionality and muscle strength as much as possible. The patient should be encouraged to participate in activities of daily living as much as can be tolerated. Active range of motion for all unaffected joints should be performed at least twice a day. If the infection is in a lower extremity, the patient may require the use of assistive devices to ambulate. Maintaining upper body strength through exercise will help the patient maintain the strength that is necessary to comfortably and safely use a walker or crutches to ambulate. It will also be important for the nurse to attend to the patient's psychosocial needs. The prolonged period of restricted activity can be frustrating to the patient and may even lead to depression. The patient may have concerns about loss of function, loss of employment, and alterations in his or her role within the family unit.

As the treatment for osteomyelitis is long-term, the patient will be discharged home on continued antibiotic therapy. If the antibiotics are still being administered intravenously, the patient and family will need to be instructed on maintenance of the venous access device and the signs and symptoms of venous inflammation that must be reported to a health care professional. The nurse must also instruct the patient and family on the importance of taking the remaining antibiotics on the prescribed time schedule, as well as the importance of completing all prescribed antibiotic therapy. Even if the patient is feeling well with no discernible symptoms of an infection, it is essential that the treatment be completed. To not complete the treatment increases the likelihood of the patient developing chronic osteomyelitis. The patient should also be instructed on how to aseptically perform any necessary dressing changes and how to safely dispose of soiled dressing materials. It may be necessary for home health nurses to visit the patient in the home to oversee management of the intravenous therapy and dressing changes.

Prior to discharge, the nurse should also instruct the patient on the importance of keeping any follow-up appointments with the physician or physical therapy. The patient should be knowledgeable about the signs and symptoms of infection and should be told to report any incidence of fever or increased pain, drainage, or swelling at the infected site.

PREVENTION OF OSTEOMYELITIS

As stated earlier, the prevention of osteomyelitis is the best treatment. Patients who have soft tissue infections should be treated promptly to decrease the likelihood of the infection spreading to the bone. Nurses should closely monitor patients who are at risk for the development of osteomyelitis, especially those with open fractures, to detect any early indications that an infection has developed at the site of injury. Patients with chronic illness, such as diabetes, should be taught the signs and symptoms of osteomyelitis and instructed to visually inspect the feet and lower extremities daily to detect any open areas.

Prophylactic antibiotics may be administered prior to orthopedic surgery to decrease the risk for osteomyelitis. Postoperative wound care should be performed using strict aseptic technique. Individuals who have had a total joint replacement may also be prescribed prophylactic antibiotics prior to invasive procedures or dental appointments. With preventive care or prompt treatment of local infections, osteomyelitis can be prevented in many patients.

SUMMARY

Osteomyelitis is a serious disorder that can lead to long-term chronic illness and disability if not diagnosed and treated promptly. Preventing osteomyelitis is the goal of care for all patients who are at risk for developing an infection of the bone. With vigilant assessment and prompt identification of potential sites of infection, the nurse can effectively help prevent the development of osteomyelitis.

EXAM QUESTIONS

CHAPTER 10
Questions 67-75

67. One risk factor for osteomyelitis is

    a. decreased calcium intake.

    b. scoliosis.

    c. closed fractures.

    d. puncture wounds.

68. Sequestrum can be best defined as

    a. an area of necrotic bone tissue.

    b. the introduction of microorganisms within the bone.

    c. the development of a sinus tract in the bone.

    d. new bone growth.

69. Chronic osteomyelitis develops when

    a. the organism causing osteomyelitis is staphylococcus aureus.

    b. infected, necrotic bone becomes sequestrum.

    c. an elderly person develops osteomyelitis.

    d. an infection has been present in the bone for 1 week.

70. One clinical manifestation of acute osteomyelitis is

    a. the presence of crepitus.

    b. insomnia with restlessness.

    c. severe pain upon movement.

    d. a draining sinus wound.

71. The primary goal of the medical management of osteomyelitis is to

    a. treat the infection as early as possible.

    b. minimize functional loss in the affected body part.

    c. prepare the patient for the likelihood of life-long therapy.

    d. encourage early mobility to prevent complications.

72. The preferred treatment for acute osteomyelitis is

    a. surgical excision of necrotic bone.

    b. aggressive antibiotic therapy.

    c. daily whirlpool therapy.

    d. administration of corticosteroids.

73. A priority nursing goal when caring for a patient with acute osteomyelitis is to

    a. improve the patient's nutritional intake.

    b. prevent spreading of the infection to others.

    c. relieve the patient's pain.

    d. encourage active range of motion in the involved extremity.

74. When caring for a patient with acute osteomyelitis, the nurse should move the affected body part by

   a. encouraging the patient to move as much as possible by himself.

   b. ensuring the body part always remains in a dependent position.

   c. applying ice packs before attempting to move the body part.

   d. supporting the body part above and below the area of infection.

75. To help prevent the development of osteomyelitis following orthopedic surgery, the nurse should

   a. monitor the patient's temperature every 4 hours.

   b. perform wound care using strict aseptic technique.

   c. obtain wound cultures 48 hours following surgery.

   d. cleanse the wound daily with hydrogen peroxide.

CHAPTER 11

CARE OF PATIENTS WITH A MUSCULOSKELETAL INJURY

CHAPTER OBJECTIVE

After completing this chapter, the reader will be able to describe the medical management and nursing care of patients who have experienced a musculoskeletal injury. Such injuries most commonly include sprains, strains, repetitive motion injuries, knee injuries, shoulder injuries, low back pain, and dislocations.

LEARNING OBJECTIVES

After studying this chapter, the reader will be able to

1. define musculoskeletal injuries.

2. indicate the pathophysiology of musculoskeletal injuries.

3. specify the medical management associated with the care of patients with a musculoskeletal injury.

4. select the nursing care associated with the care of patients with a musculoskeletal injury.

OVERVIEW

Musculoskeletal injuries that result in damage to the soft tissues of the musculoskeletal system are some of the most common injuries. These injuries are frequently due to hazards in the home environment, occupational risks, and sports or physical fitness activities. These common injuries result in the loss of many days of productivity annually in the United States. Health education in the community could decrease a number of these injuries. Nurses have a responsibility to educate the public about accident prevention and safe participation in physical fitness and sports activities. This chapter will address the medical management and nursing care of some of the most common musculoskeletal injuries that occur in the United States.

STRAINS AND SPRAINS

Strains and sprains are common injuries. A strain is a pull or tear in a skeletal muscle. It is frequently caused by overuse or overstretching of the muscle, and it may be acute due to sudden trauma or chronic in nature due to repetitive motion. Tendons can also suffer a strain (McCance & Mourad, 2000). Twisting or wrenching motions frequently lead to a strain.

A patient who experiences a strain will feel a muscle spasm and pain. There will be local tenderness at the muscle upon movement. Continued use of the muscle will aggravate the discomfort. The more serious strains will also exhibit edema, ecchymosis (bruising), and a decrease in function (Roberts, 2001).

A sprain is an injury to a ligament caused by a wrenching or twisting motion that overextends the ligament (Liddel, 2000b). The ankle is the most common joint that experiences a sprain. The symptoms experienced by the patient will depend upon the degree of the sprain. A first degree sprain is relatively mild, with only a few fibers being torn. As a result the patient experiences only mild discomfort and a slight swelling. A second degree sprain involves disruption of over half of the ligament fibers. Patients who experience a second degree sprain will experience more swelling and pain. A third degree sprain indicates that the ligament has been completely torn. The patient will experience acute pain and swelling as well as loss of function. In the case of a third degree sprain, the patient may actually experience an avulsion fracture to the bone, with a portion of the bone pulled away by the torn ligament (Ruda, 2000b).

The treatment for strains and sprains is relatively similar and dependent upon the degree of injury suffered. An x-ray is frequently taken to examine the body structure for injury to the bone. Initial treatment of a strain or sprain consists of RICE, which is an easy to remember acronym for treatment intervention (see Table 11–1).

TABLE 11–1: TREATMENT OF STRAINS AND SPRAINS
Rest
Ice
Compression
Elevation

The patient is instructed to *rest* the affected joint to avoid any further injury to the tissues. During the first 24 to 48 hours following the injury, *ice* is applied to the injury for intervals of 20–30 minutes. Following the application of ice for 20–30 minutes, the ice compress is removed to prevent tissue damage. After about 15 minutes, the ice compress can be reapplied. Ice promotes vasoconstriction in the area ,which helps decrease the swelling and bleeding into the tissue. An elastic bandage is wrapped over the injured joint to provide *compression* and support to limit swelling. The nurse should check the bandage frequently to be sure that it is not con-

stricting circulation, and it should be removed at frequent intervals to inspect the skin. The injured part is also kept *elevated* above the level of the heart at all times to decrease swelling. Following the acute phase of the injury (first 24–48 hours), ice is discontinued, and heat applications may be used intermittently (30 minutes) to promote vasodilation and decrease pain from muscle spasms. Heat is usually applied about four times a day (Liddel, 2000b).

Mild sprains and strains usually take about 3–5 days to heal; a second degree injury may take 1–2 weeks (Ruda, 2000b). During the recovery phase, it is essential that the patient continue to limit activity and not overuse the joint; overuse will result in an extended recovery period. Third degree sprains may require surgical intervention with the application of a cast or brace following surgery. It can take up to 6 weeks for healing to occur.

REPETITIVE MOTION INJURIES

The incidence of repetitive motion injuries or repetitive strain injuries (RSI) is rapidly increasing. RSI results from repeated movements that strain tendons, muscles, and ligaments. Tiny tears in these soft tissues develop, leading to inflammation (Ruda, 2000b). Over a period of time, if these tears are not allowed to heal, scarring occurs with consequent constriction of blood vessels and nerves and the development of chronic pain.

The increase in repetitive motion injuries can be linked to the increased use of computers in the workplace and for recreation. In addition to the repetitive motions involved in keyboarding, poorly designed workstations are another cause of injury. The areas most commonly affected by injury from the repetitive motions caused by computer use are the hands, wrists, forearms, shoulders, and the neck (Ruda, 2000b). Anyone with an occupation that requires repetitive use of a joint is at risk for RSI.

One specific condition that is caused by repetitive motion injury is carpal tunnel syndrome. Carpal tunnel syndrome is caused by ligaments at the wrist compressing the median nerve; it is associated with occupations that require repetitive wrist movement such as computer operators, beauticians, carpenters, etc. Women are most often affected by the syndrome, and it usually develops in the dominant hand (Marek, 1999b).

The signs and symptoms of carpal tunnel syndrome include pain, numbness, weakness, and difficulty performing fine motor movements in the affected hand. The pain may be more bothersome at night, and many people report being awakened by the discomfort. If the condition goes untreated, the patient may develop thenar atrophy, which is atrophy of the muscle located at the base of the thumb (Ruda, 2000b).

Diagnosis of carpal tunnel syndrome is made based upon the patient's symptoms. A Phalen's test may also be conducted to diagnose the condition. This involves acutely flexing the wrist for 60 seconds to see if the symptoms can be elicited. If they are, this is considered to be a positive Phalen's test. A positive Tinel's sign occurs when the examiner taps the area of the median nerve and causes paresthesia (Marek, 1999b).

Treatment of carpal tunnel syndrome includes the use of wrist splints to promote rest of the joint and relief of the inflammation. Nonsteroidal anti-inflammatory medications may decrease pain and a corticosteroid injection directly into the joint can also provide relief. If these conservative measures do not work, the patient may need to undergo surgery to achieve decompression of the median nerve. This is usually an outpatient surgery that requires the patient to wear a splint for 2–3 weeks postoperatively. Immediately following surgery, the neurovascular status of the affected hand must be assessed every hour for the first 24 hours. The nurse will instruct the patient on what signs and symptoms should be reported to the surgeon.

Because of the increase in RSI, one of the nurse's most important roles is to engage in patient education and health promotion activities. The use of proper body mechanics and an increased awareness of health promotion activities in the work environment that can decrease occupational hazards can effectively decrease the incidence of this health problem.

KNEE LIGAMENT AND MENISCUS INJURIES

Ligament Injuries

One category of common sports-related injuries is those that occur to the ligaments and meniscus of the knees. Ligaments provide joint support and stability. The most common knee ligament injury is a tear of the anterior cruciate ligament (ACL), which occurs as a result of hyperextension of the knee and simultaneous twisting of the femur on a firmly planted foot (Liddel, 2000b). ACL injuries most commonly occur in individuals between the ages of 15 and 44 (Childs, 2002). Football, basketball, soccer, and skiing account for many of these injuries.

When the ACL is torn, the patient will complain of acute pain, difficulty ambulating, and knee joint instability. Swelling will also develop in the joint (Marek, 1999b). The treatment of the injury will depend upon the severity. Conservative, nonsurgical treatment of the injury consists of RICE, the use of analgesics and non-steroidal anti-inflammatory medications, and the application of a brace to rest and stabilize the joint.

If it appears that nonsurgical treatment will not be effective, the patient may undergo surgical repair of the tear as an outpatient. Arthroscopic surgery will be conducted. Neurovascular assessments, wound care, and the prevention of infection are immediate postoperative care goals. Physical therapy will also be required following surgery to aid the restoration of range of motion in the knee. The rehabilitation of the knee may take anywhere from 6–12 months following surgery (Liddel, 2000b).

Collateral ligaments in the knee are also subject to tear. Typically, this injury occurs when the patient has a foot planted solidly on the ground and is struck either medially or laterally, stretching the collateral ligament. Signs and symptoms of a collateral ligament injury includes acute pain, loss of ability to ambulate unassisted, and instability of the knee. Treatment and nursing care are similar that that of an ACL tear.

Meniscus Injuries

The meniscus cartilage is present in the knees between the tibia and the femoral condyles. Meniscal injuries can occur whenever there is twisting of the knee or repetitive bending that results in a tear in the cartilage. Typically, this type of injury is related to sports activities, and it is common to see a meniscus injury along with a ligament injury. A torn meniscus can result in pain and tenderness. The patient most likely will report hearing or feeling a click within the knee upon movement. The knee may also lock, or it may feel like it is going to "give way." This feeling of joint instability is due to the torn meniscus being loose within the knee joint and preventing full extension of the knee joint (Liddel, 2000b).

Diagnosis of a meniscus injury is made by an MRI or an arthroscopy (Andres, Mears, & Wenz, 2001). Treatment consists of surgical removal of the torn cartilage through an arthroscopy conducted as an outpatient procedure. After the surgery, the knee will be immobilized with a splint to protect it, and the patient will use crutches to ambulate. Most patients can return to normal activity within a few days of surgery. One potential complication following surgery is joint effusion. If this occurs, the physician will aspirate fluid from the joint (Ruda, 2000b).

ROTATOR CUFF INJURIES

Rotator cuff injuries may be acute or chronic in nature. Acute injuries are usually due to trauma, falls, or sports injuries. Chronic problems are most often related to repetitive motion stress and injury. The rotator cuff consists of four muscles: supraspinatus, infraspinatus, teres minor, and subscapularis. The functions of these muscles are to stabilize the humerus head and rotate the humerus (Ruda, 2000b).

A torn rotator cuff causes pain and limited mobility to develop in the shoulder. The patient will experience limited range of motion in the joint and may be unable to abduct the arm and shoulder. A torn cuff is diagnosed with a MRI. An arthrogram can also be used to diagnose the extent of the tear.

Treatment of a torn rotator cuff may be either conservative or surgical. Conservative treatment consists of rest, ice, and non-steroidal anti-inflammatory medications, followed by physical therapy to regain the joint's range of motion. Corticosteroid injections in the joint may also be used. If this treatment is not successful, then surgical correction of the tear will be performed through an arthroscope. Postoperatively, the shoulder will be immobilized. The nurse will check the neurovascular status of the affected arm periodically during the immediate postoperative phase. Analgesics will be administered to treat shoulder pain. Shoulder exercises should be started a few days after surgery, and physical therapy will gradually progress to resistive exercises. It will take about 6 months to 1 year for the patient to regain full use of the shoulder (Ruda, 2000b).

LOW BACK PAIN

It is estimated that low back pain has affected about 80% of the adults living in the United States at some point in time. It is one of the most common occupational injuries and is costly in terms of lost work productivity and medical expenses (Ruda, 2000b).

Risk factors associated with muscle strain that leads to low back pain include improper body mechanics, poor posture, obesity, smoking, sedentary lifestyles, and prolonged sitting, stress, and repetitive lifting (Ruda, 2000b). Low back pain can also develop as a result of a number of physical problems, including arthritis, intervertebral disk problems, osteoporosis, abdominal tumors, and bone cancer metastasis (Liddel, 2000b). Diagnostic tests will be necessary to rule out these other physical health problems and determine the cause of the back pain. Mechanical strain of the paravertebral muscles is the most common cause of lower back pain (Ruda, 2000b).

The lumbosacral area is commonly affected by pain due to the fact that it is the most flexible portion of the spine, bears the majority of the body's weight, is somewhat mechanically unstable, and has a number of nerve roots that are susceptible to injury (Ruda, 2000b).

Clinical manifestations of lower back strain include pain. The pain may be acute or chronic in nature. Pain lasting longer than 3 months is considered chronic. The patient may complain of radiating pain down the leg, which is indicative of nerve involvement. Pain radiating down the back of the leg is referred to as sciatica. The patient may complain of muscle spasms. Fatigue may also be present. If the patient is asked to perform straight leg raises, this may elicit sciatica pain (Liddel, 2000b).

Conservative treatment is implemented on an outpatient basis and consists of pharmacological intervention. Analgesics are prescribed to treat the pain. Muscle relaxants are prescribed to relieve muscle spasms. Non-steroidal anti-inflammatory medications are used to treat inflammation. If the pain is severe, bed rest may also be prescribed. Heat or cold therapy may also be applied to relieve muscle spasms. As the pain improves, physical therapy

may be implemented to help strengthen back muscles and to teach the patient proper body mechanics.

The nurse plays a prominent role in patient teaching as well. Table 11–2 describes the patient education related to low back problems. The nurse should encourage the patient to make the necessary lifestyle adjustments to successfully treat low back pain.

TABLE 11-2: LOW BACK PROBLEMS

Do Not
- Lean forward without bending knees
- Lift anything above level of elbows
- Stand in one position for prolonged time
- Sleep on abdomen or on back or side with legs out straight
- Exercise without consulting health care provider if having severe pain
- Exceed prescribed amount and type of exercises without consulting health care provider

Do
- Prevent lower back from straining forward by placing a foot on a step or stool during prolonged standing
- Sleep in a side-lying position with knees and hips bent
- Sleep on back with a lift under knees and legs or on back with 10-inch-high pillow under knees to flex hips and knees
- Sit in a chair with knees higher than hips and support arms on chair or knees
- Exercise 15 min in the morning and 15 min in the evening regularly; begin exercises with a 2- or 3-min warm-up period by moving arms and legs, by alternately relaxing and tightening muscles; exercise slowly with smooth movements as directed by a physical therapist
- Avoid chilling during and after exercising
- Maintain appropriate body weight
- use a lumbar roll or pillow for sitting

From Lewis, S., Heitkemper, M., & Dirksen, S. (2000). *Medical-surgical nursing: Assessment and management of clinical problems* (5th ed., p. 1806). St. Louis, MO: Mosby. Reprinted with permission from Elsevier.

JOINT DISLOCATIONS

A joint dislocation is a traumatic condition in which the articular surfaces of the joint, or the joint ends, are no longer in alignment with each other. A subluxation is a condition in which the joint is partially dislocated. The elbow, shoulder, wrist, finger, knee, and hip are the joints that are most prone to dislocation (McCance & Mourad, 2000).

Total or partial dislocations are most commonly caused by trauma. Falls, motor vehicle accidents and sports activities are some leading causes of dislocations. However, dislocations may also be a congenital problem.

Dislocations may be associated with a fracture due to the trauma that usually occurs. Not only is the bone disrupted, but surrounding soft tissues, blood vessels, and nerves may also be injured. If circulation to surrounding tissues is disrupted, ischemia may develop. If not treated promptly with circulation restored, permanent damage may be inflicted on surrounding structures. For this reason, a dislocation can be an orthopedic emergency (McCance & Mourad, 2000).

Signs and symptoms of a dislocation or subluxation of a joint includes joint deformity, pain, loss of function, and swelling. The length of the extremity may be affected as well. The patient's discomfort is acute. Treatment of the patient includes immobilization of the dislocated joint so that further damage cannot occur prior to correction of the dislocation. The dislocation will be reduced, either under a regional or general anesthetic. The patient will require analgesics and muscle relaxants to promote comfort. The joint will also be immobilized to provide rest and stability to the joint and to promote healing in the surrounding structures (Ruda, 2000b).

Nursing care of the patient following treatment for a dislocation includes neurovascular assessments before and after surgery. Pain control will be a primary goal. Immobilization of the affected joint will also be a priority nursing goal. The patient will gradually regain mobility of the joint through an exercise program. The joint may be predisposed to future dislocations, so the nurse must teach the patient how to protect the joint from reinjury and how to correctly apply any immobilizing devices that are prescribed for the patient's use.

SUMMARY

Musculoskeletal injuries are common. In the majority of the cases, the patient will be treated in an ambulatory setting and discharged soon after care has been received. The nurse's role is primarily one of preparing the patient preoperatively for any diagnostic and surgical procedures and providing the immediate postoperative care. Because of the patient's quick discharge from the health care setting, patient education for care in the home setting is an essential nursing function. Prior to discharge, the patient and family members should know how to assess for potential neurovascular complications and signs of infection. The patient should also be instructed in the use of any prescribed medications, how to correctly use immobilization or ambulation devices, and when to return to the health care provider for follow-up appointments. It is also important for the nurse to emphasize when the patient should seek further medical advice. Finally, since many of these injuries are preventable, public education on selected health promotion and safety issues is another responsibility of the nurse.

CASE STUDY

You are working in the walk-in clinic when A.H., a 20 year-old female comes into the clinic complaining of sharp pain in the left ankle. She tells you that she was playing volleyball when she "twisted" her ankle after jumping up to "spike" the ball over the net. Her ankle is swollen, and she has difficulty bearing weight on it due to the pain. The physician diagnoses an ankle sprain. A.H. is told to not bear weight on her ankle for the next 2-3 days and to use crutches to help her ambulate. It is your responsibility to provide discharge instructions to her.

Answer the following case study questions, writing your responses on a separate sheet of paper. Compare your responses to the answers that are located at the end of the chapter.

1. During this initial phase of A.H.'s injury, what should you instruct her to do to decrease pain and swelling in the ankle?

2. What treatment should A.H. be instructed to initiate for 24–48 hours post-injury?

3. Describe safety instructions for the use of cold and heat applications that you will teach A.H.

4. What important patient safety tips should you give A.H. when teaching her how to walk with her crutches?

Answers to Case Study

1. A.H. should be taught the RICE treatment, which stands for: Rest, Ice, Compression, and Elevation. She should be instructed to rest the ankle, apply ice, maintain a compression bandage in place, and elevate the extremity above the level of the heart. The ice is applied for 20–30 minutes and then removed for 15 minutes to avoid tissue damage. After a 15 minute rest, the ice compress can be reapplied.

2. Following the initial phase of the injury (24–48 hours), ice therapy is discontinued and heat therapy is applied to decrease muscle spasms, promote comfort, and support the healing process. The heat is usually applied about 4 times a day for approximately 30 minutes each time.

3. Safety precautions that should be implemented when applying either cold or heat therapy include first carefully inspecting the skin in the affected area and noting any alterations in skin integrity. You will carefully assess the condition of A.H.'s skin following the treatment as well. Heat therapy should not be applied to any area that is actively bleeding, and cold therapy should not be applied to any area that is edematous. All equipment should be carefully inspected to ensure safe functioning. A.H. should be instructed not to adjust any temperature settings and to report immediately any feelings of discomfort. All treatments should be carefully timed, adhering to the prescribed length of time for the therapy. Heat therapy should be applied for limited periods of time to avoid reflex vasoconstriction. Cold therapy is applied for limited time periods to avoid tissue damage and reflex vasodilation. The therapy is documented, including the length of time it was applied, the appearance of the area following the therapy, and the patient's response to the treatment.

4. A.H. must be taught the three-point gait, as she is not allowed to bear weight on the right ankle. She should be instructed to wear sturdy walking shoes with low heels. A.H. should be taught how to inspect her crutches for loose screws and bolts and to check the rubber tips. It is important that A.H. be instructed not to lean on the crutch axilla pads, as that can lead to brachial nerve pressure. Other safety precautions include how to ascend and descend stairs.

EXAM QUESTIONS

CHAPTER 11
Questions 76-79

76. A sprain is defined as a

    a. tear in skeletal muscle.

    b. bruised bone.

    c. overextended ligament.

    d. torn tendon.

77. Carpal tunnel syndrome is caused by compression of the

    a. ulnar nerve.

    b. radial nerve.

    c. brachial nerve.

    d. median nerve.

78. A patient who has torn his anterior cruciate ligament should

    a. apply a heating pad.

    b. apply ice.

    c. receive an intra-articular injection of corticosteroids.

    d. maintain the knee in a flexed position.

79. The nurse providing postoperative care for a patient who had surgery for a rotator cuff tear should give priority to

    a. neurovascular checks of the affected arm.

    b. application of ice to the surgical site.

    c. elevation of the arm above the level of the heart.

    d. administration of intravenous antibiotics.

CHAPTER 12

CARE OF THE PATIENT WITH ARTHRITIS

CHAPTER OBJECTIVE

After completing this chapter, the reader will be able to describe the nursing care of patients who have arthritis. Rheumatoid arthritis, osteoarthritis (degenerative joint disease) and gout will be discussed.

LEARNING OBJECTIVES

After studying this chapter, the reader will be able to

1. identify the etiology and risk factors for the development of arthritis.

2. differentiate the two major types of arthritis: rheumatoid arthritis and osteoarthritis.

3. indicate the pathophysiology of inflammation and degeneration as it relates to arthritis.

4. specify the clinical manifestations of arthritis.

5. select the medical management and nursing care of patients with arthritis.

OVERVIEW

The term *arthritis* means inflammation of the joint. There are over 100 different types of arthritis disorders that affect 40 million people in the United States alone (Marek, 1999b). Arthritis is one of the most common chronic disorders in the United States. The decreased productivity, the loss of wages, and the health care costs associated with arthritis amount to billions of dollars annually.

There are 13 groups of joint disease recognized by the American Rheumatism Association. These diseases can be classified as either a noninflammatory joint disease or an inflammatory joint disease (McCance & Mourad, 2000). Rheumatoid arthritis and gout are inflammatory joint diseases. Osteoarthritis is a noninflammatory joint disease. Because of these underlying differences in the pathophysiology of each disease, there are some specific differences in the medical management and nursing care associated with each condition. This chapter will discuss the medical management and nursing care of patients with rheumatoid arthritis, osteoarthritis, and gout.

RHEUMATOID ARTHRITIS

Rheumatoid arthritis (RA) is a chronic, systemic, autoimmune disease that is characterized by inflammation of the synovial membrane and articular cartilage of the joints (McCance & Mourad, 2000). Since it is a systemic disease, the effects of the disease are not limited to joints. Rheumatoid arthritis most often affects the joints, but it can affect other connective tissues as well. The majority of individuals who have RA are women who are over 30 years of age (Bush, 2000). Rheumatoid arthritis is characterized by periods of remission and exacerbation. There is no cure.

Etiology and Risk Factors

There is no known cause for RA. There are several theories that are being studied. One is that RA is due to an infectious organism that has yet to be identified. Another theory is that RA is an autoimmunity disorder triggered by a virus. This is the most likely possibility. Another theory suggests that there is a genetic predisposition in some cases to the development of RA (Bush, 2000). There are no specific risk factors associated with RA.

Pathophysiology

RA develops in four stages. All of the damage that occurs in the joint is the result of the inflammatory process and the resulting formation of scar tissue. In the first stage, inflammation of the synovial membrane begins. As part of the inflammatory response, the synovial membrane thickens and more synovial fluid is produced. In the second stage of the disease, an inflammatory granulation tissue, known as pannus, grows over the articular cartilage and invades other surfaces within the joint. In the third stage of the disease, the pannus is gradually replaced by scar tissue that fills up the joint space. This nonfunctioning scar tissue is tough and fibrous, and it leads to a loss of function in the joint and the development of deformities. In the fourth and final stage, the fibrous tissue begins to calcify, eventually resulting in an immobile, or ankylosed, joint (Bush, 2000). The patient is left with a nonfunctioning, painful joint.

Clinical Manifestations

The signs and symptoms of RA can be divided into those that occur within the joint and those that occur systemically. The onset of the disease is usually insidious. The patient may initially have some vague, general complaints, which are nonspecific, such as fatigue, fever, lack of appetite, weight loss, and aching and stiffness (McCance & Mourad, 2000).

Gradually, localized joint manifestations begin to appear. The joints become painful and tender to touch, with swelling and a feeling of warmth in

them. The joints are affected in a bilaterally symmetrical manner, and the smaller joints of the hands and feet are often the first to be affected. The larger, weight-bearing joints are usually affected later. The patient will begin to notice joint stiffness in the morning when getting out of bed or after prolonged periods of immobility. This stiffness lasts 30 minutes or longer.

Over a period of time, the interphalangeal joints and metacarpal joints begin to swell and become deformed, taking on a spindle shape (Bush, 2000). The swelling in the joints is due to inflammatory exudate and will feel "boggy" when palpated (McCance & Mourad, 2000). Other deformities in the joints develop as well, eventually leading to disability. See Figure 12–1 for an illustration of common deformities associated with RA (Bush, 2000). As the joints become immobile, the muscles surrounding the joints begin to atrophy.

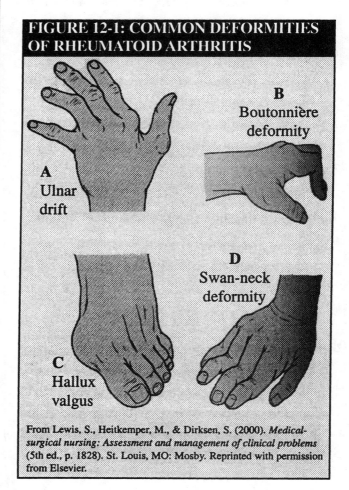

FIGURE 12-1: COMMON DEFORMITIES OF RHEUMATOID ARTHRITIS

A Ulnar drift

B Boutonnière deformity

C Hallux valgus

D Swan-neck deformity

From Lewis, S., Heitkemper, M., & Dirksen, S. (2000). *Medical-surgical nursing: Assessment and management of clinical problems* (5th ed., p. 1828). St. Louis, MO: Mosby. Reprinted with permission from Elsevier.

Outside of the joints, rheumatoid nodules develop and may be present in any connective tissue. Approximately 25–50% of the people with RA develop rheumatoid nodules (see Figure 12–2). These nodules are firm and nontender; they are most commonly found in subcutaneous tissue on the elbows and fingers, although they can form anywhere on the body. These nodules can also invade the pericardium, heart valves, lung tissue, and spleen, leading to inflammatory problems in these organs. The eyes can also be affected by the nodules, leading to acute glaucoma (Bush, 2000). Organ damage can be extensive.

FIGURE 12-2: RHEUMATOID ARTHRITIS OF THE HAND

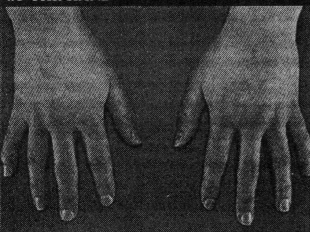

Early stage

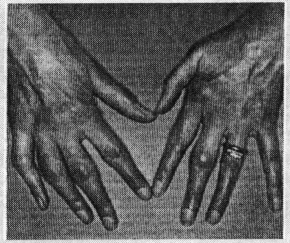

Moderate involvement

From Lewis, S., Heitkemper, M., & Dirksen, S. (2000). *Medical-surgical nursing: Assessment and management of clinical problems* (5th ed., p. 1828). St. Louis, MO: Mosby. Reprinted with permission from Elsevier.

It must be remembered that RA is a disease characterized by remission and exacerbation. It can be mild or it can be progressively debilitating. Patients can manifest the signs and symptoms in a number of different ways, and the disease is unpredictable.

Diagnosis

RA is diagnosed based upon symptoms and laboratory tests that are seldom conclusive. The American Rheumatism Association has identified diagnostic criteria for RA (see Table 12–1). The patient must exhibit four or more criteria for a diagnosis of RA, and the first four criteria listed in the table must be present for at least 6 weeks.

TABLE 12–1: DIAGNOSTIC CRITERIA FOR RHEUMATOID ARTHRITIS (AMERICAN RHEUMATISM ASSOCIATION)*

Morning stiffness

Arthritis in 3 or more joints

Arthritis in hands

Symmetrical arthritis

Presence of rheumatoid nodules

Positive serum rheumatoid factor test

Radiographic changes

* The patient must exhibit four or more criteria for a diagnosis of RA, and the first four criteria listed in the table must be present for at least 6 weeks.

From McCance & Mourad. (2000). Alterations of musculoskeletal function. In S.E. Huether, & K.L. McCance (Eds.). *Understanding pathophysiology* (2nd ed.), (pp. 1031–1073). St. Louis: Mosby, Inc.

In addition to the criteria cited by the American Rheumatism Association, there are other laboratory tests that may be positive but do not provide a definitive diagnosis. Many patients with RA will have an elevated erythrocyte sedimentation rate (ESR). Antinuclear antibodies and lupus cell tests may be positive in some. It is common for patients with RA to exhibit a moderate form of anemia.

Synovial fluid may be aspirated from the joints for analysis. There is an increased volume and increased turbidity in the fluid; the viscosity is decreased. White blood cell count in the fluid will be elevated. X-rays may not show any changes until the later stages of the disease when the cartilage destruction, deformity, and narrowed joint space become evident (Bush, 2000).

Medical Management

The mainstay of the medical management of RA is drug therapy. For years, large doses of aspirin and nonsteroidal anti-inflammatories (NSAIDs) were the main drugs used to treat RA. In recent years, however, the treatment of RA with drugs has become increasingly aggressive in an effort to delay progression of the disease to its later stages.

It is now becoming common to see disease-modifying anti-rheumatic drugs (DMARDs) prescribed earlier in the course of the disease (Marek, 1999b).

The physician will usually start drug therapy with the least toxic medication that is effective (Bush, 2000). For many patients who have mild symptoms and little to no detected joint changes, the first line of drug therapy remains the NSAIDs. Aspirin is still used as well in large doses. There are many NSAIDs available on the market; the physician will try different drugs until an effective one is found for the patient. It usually takes about 2–3 weeks before effectiveness can be determined (Marek, 1999b). Some of the newer NSAIDs, COX-2 inhibitors, have proven particularly effective for some patients (Bush, 2000).

If the NSAIDs and salycilates are not effective, the next line of drugs is the DMARDs. These can be used alone or in combination with the NSAIDs. Two of the more commonly prescribed DMARDs are hydroxychloroquine (Plaquenil), which is an antimalarial drug, and methotrexate, which is an immunosuppressive drug. If methotrexate or hydroxychloroquine are not effective, gold therapy may be implemented. Azathioprine and D-penicillamine may be used if the previous drugs are not

effective. If none of the previous drugs have proven successful at treating the patient, other immunosuppressive drugs such as Cytoxan® (cyclophosphamide) can be prescribed (Marek, 1999b). Immunomodulators, such as leflunomide and etanercept, may also be prescribed if other drug therapy has proven ineffective.

Steroids also have a role in treating RA. Corticosteroids may be given for short-term use while the physician is experimenting to find other effective medications. They may also be administered during acute exacerbations of the disease. And finally, intra-articular injections may be used to treat particularly painful individual joints. Long-term use of steroid therapy is contraindicated (Bush, 2000).

Drug therapy for each patient is highly individualized. The primary goal of the drug therapy is to relieve pain. Treatment of RA with effective drug therapy can delay the progression of joint destruction, thus maintaining joint function and a higher quality of life for the patient. Table 12–2 summarizes current drug therapy for RA and describes nursing considerations related to each drug category. A primary responsibility of the nurse is patient education. Patients should be informed of drug dosage, actions, side effects, and any potential interactions with other drugs.

In addition to drug therapy, the patient will also engage in exercise programs and, in general, must develop good health habits. If joint function is affected, physical therapy and occupational therapy will help the patient to adjust the performance of activities of daily living and maintain independence. If drug therapy is not effective in treating the patient, surgical reconstruction of the joint through joint replacement may be possible.

Nursing Care

The nurse assesses the patient for signs and symptoms of RA and determines how the disease has affected the patient's ability to participate in the normal activities of daily living. Fatigue, anorexia,

TABLE 12-2: MEDICATIONS COMMONLY USED TO TREAT RHEUMATOID ARTHRITIS (1 OF 3)

Medications	Uses/Effects	Side Effects	Monitoring
Aspirin and other nonsteroidal anti-inflammatory drugs (NSAIDs) Examples: • Plain aspirin • Buffered aspirin • Ibuprofen (Advil,* Motrin IB) • Ketoprofen (Orudis) • Naproxen (Naprosyn) • Celecoxib (Celebrex) • Rofecoxib (Vioxx)	• Used to reduce pain, swelling, and inflammation, allowing patients to move more easily and carry out normal activities • Generally part of early and continuing therapy	• Upset stomach • Tendency to bruise easily • Fluid retention (NSAIDs other than aspirin) • Ulcers • Possible kidney and liver damage (rare)	Patients should have periodic blood tests.
Medications	**Uses/Effects**	**Side Effects**	**Monitoring**
Disease-modifying antirheumatic drugs (DMARDs) (also called slow-acting antirheumatic drugs [SAARDs] or second-line drugs) Examples: • Gold, injectable or oral (Myochrysine, Ridaura) • Antimalarials, such as hydroxychloroquine (Plaquenil) • Penicillamine (Cuprimine, Depen) • Sulfasalazine (Azulfidine)	• Used to alter the course of the disease and prevent joint and cartilage destruction • May produce significant improvement for many patients • Exactly how they work still unknown • Generally take a few weeks or months to have an effect • Patients may use several over the course of the disease	• Toxicity is an issue--DMARDs can have serious side effects: Gold-skin rash, mouth sores, upset stomach, kidney problems, low blood count • Antimalarials - upset stomach, eye problems (rare) • Penicillamine-- skin rashes, upset stomach, blood abnormalities, kidney problems • Sulfasalazine - upset stomach	Patients should be monitored carefully for continued effectiveness of medication and for side effects: • Gold-blood and urine test monthly; more often in early use of drug • Antimalarials - eye exam every 6 months • Penicillamine - blood and urine test monthly; more often in early use of drug • Sulfasalazine - periodic blood and urine tests

joint pain, and stiffness will affect the person's ability to fully participate in meaningful activities. The nurse also assesses the patient's knowledge of the disease and treatment management. Education is important to help the patient learn how to manage the disease. The goals of nursing care include decreasing pain, maintaining joint function, managing fatigue, maintaining mobility, and educating the patient about self-care and disease management. Since RA is a systemic disease, the nurse develops

TABLE 12-2: MEDICATIONS COMMONLY USED TO TREAT RHEUMATOID ARTHRITIS (2 OF 3)

Medications	Uses/Effects	Side Effects	Monitoring
Immuno-suppressants (also considered DMARDs) Examples: • Methotrexate (Rheumatrex) • Azathioprine (Imuran) • Cyclosporine (Sandimmune, Neoral) • Lefluomide (Arava)	• Used to restrain the overly active immune system, which is key to the disease process • Same concerns as with other DMARDs: potential toxicity and diminishing effectiveness over time • Methotrexate can result in rapid improvement; appears to be very effective • Azathioprine - first used in higher doses in cancer chemo-therapy and organ transplantation; used in patients who have not responded to other drugs; used in combination therapy • Cyclosporine-- first used in organ transplantation to prervent rejection; used in patients who have not responded to other drugs • Leflunomide-- reduces signs and symptoms as well as retards structural damage to joints caused by arthritis	Toxicity is an issue- immunosuppressants can have serious side effects: • Methotrexate - upset stomach, potential liver problems, low white blood cell count • Azathioprine - potential blood abnormalities, low white blood cell count, possible increased cancer risk • Cyclosporine - high blood pressure, hair growth, tremors, loss of kidney function • Leflunomide - diarrhea, skin rashes, hair loss, liver problems	Patients should be monitored carefully for continued effectiveness of medication and for side effects: • Methotrexate - regular blood tests, including liver function test; baseline chest x ray • Azathioprine - regular blood and liver function tests • Cyclosporine - regular blood tests, including kidney function, and blood pressure • Leflunomide - regular blood tests, including liver function tests

TABLE 12-2: MEDICATIONS COMMONLY USED TO TREAT RHEUMATOID ARTHRITIS (3 OF 3)

Medications	Uses/Effects	Side Effects	Monitoring
Corticosteroids (also known as glucocorticoids) Examples: • Prednisone (Deltasone, Orasone) • Methylprednisolone (Medrol)	• Used for their anti-inflammatory and immuno-suppressive effects • Given either in pill form or as an injection into a joint • Dramatic improvements in a very short time • Potential for serious side effects, especially at high doses • Often used early while waiting for DMARDs to work • Also used for severe flares and when the disease does not respond to NSAIDs and DMARDs	• Osteoporosis • Mood changes • Fragile skin, easy bruising • Fluid retention • Weight gain • Muscle weakness • Onset or worsening of diabetes • Cataracts • Increased risk of infection • Hypertension (high blood pressure)	Patients should be monitored carefully for continued effectiveness of medication and for side effects.
Biologic Response Modifiers Example: • Etanercept (Enbrel)	• Effective in patients with mild to moderate rheumatoid arthitis who have failed other drug therapies and, in addition, in patients with juvenile rheumatoid arthritis. Given as a twice-a-week injection into the skin	• Skin reactions at injection sites, infection, headaches	Patients should be monitored closely for signs of infection.

* Brand names included in this booklet are provided as examples only, and their inclusion does not mean that these products are endorsed by the National Institutes of Health or any other Government agency. Also, if a particular brand name is not mentioned, this does not mean or imply that the product is unsatisfactory.

From National Institute of Arthritis and Musculoskeletal and Skin Diseases (NIAMS) (1999). *Handout on Health: Rheumatoid Arthritis.* Retrieved April 2, 2004 from http://www.niams.nih.gov/hi/topics/arthritis/rahandout.htm#ra_5

a plan of care that promotes healthy living habits, including good nutrition and good sleep habits.

In addition to administering the drug therapy and ensuring that the patient understands the regimen, there are additional nursing interventions that can be taken to help increase the patient's comfort. If the patient is overweight, a weight reduction diet should be recommended to decrease the stress that is placed on the joints by the extra weight. There is no particular diet for the patient with RA to follow; however, the patient should be encouraged to have a well-balanced diet with adequate protein and vitamins.

Assistive devices, such as braces and splints, can be used by the patient to rest individual joints that are acutely inflamed. Crutches and walkers can be used to decrease weight-bearing on painful joints, and to provide support. Other adaptive devices can be used to help the patient dress, eat, and bath independently. The nurse reinforces the instructions that have been provided by physical therapists and occupational therapists on how to use these devices appropriately.

The application of heat and cold also has a role in the treatment of RA. Heat may be used to relieve stiffness, muscle spasms, and decrease pain. Heating pads, paraffin baths, and warm compresses may all provide comfort. The patient should be instructed on how to use heat applications safely and should be reminded that heat applications should be limited to no more than 20 minutes at a time to prevent skin damage (Pigg, 2000). If a joint is acutely inflamed, heat may not be comfortable to the patient; rather, applications of cold therapy provide a local anesthetic effect to the joint while helping to decrease muscle spasms and soothe the pain. Again, the patient should be taught the safe application of cold therapy, including the importance of removing the cold application after an interval of about 20 minutes to avoid injuring the skin.

The patient should be taught to get a minimum of eight hours of sleep every night and to plan rest periods during the day to combat the chronic fatigue that

is associated with RA. Tips on how to conserve energy while protecting the joints will also be beneficial to the patient. Since RA is a systemic disease, it is important that the patient rest the body, not just the affected joints. Patients should also be taught the importance of proper positioning while lying in bed. The patient should be sure <u>not</u> to assume any position or use pillows in any manner that might promote flexion contractures in the joints. This may be difficult for some patients, as it is natural to want to assume a position of least discomfort. Positioning the joints in a flexed position is frequently more comfortable than maintaining them in a position of extension. However, allowing patients to assume a position of flexion promotes the development of flexion contractures. Splints may be helpful in maintaining the fingers and wrists in an extended position at night. A firm mattress and small, flat pillows for the head will also help maintain alignment. The nurse should also instruct the patient in the importance of gently putting each joint through a full range of motion each day to help preserve function (Pigg, 2000).

The nurse should also attend to the psychosocial needs of the patient. The potential loss of independence and the body image changes can affect the person's self-esteem levels. Being diagnosed with a chronic illness may also have financial and occupational implications. RA support groups can be found in most communities and can be a source of great support to patients. The nurse should refer the patient to any community resources that may be beneficial to the patient.

OSTEOARTHRITIS

Osteoarthritis, also known as degenerative joint disease, is the most common of all joint disorders (Pigg, 2000). In contrast to RA, it is not a systemic, inflammatory disease. Rather it is a disease where the primary process is degeneration of the articular cartilage. The differences between RA and OA are captured in Table 12–3.

TABLE 12-3: COMPARISON OF RHEUMATOID ARTHRITIS AND OSTEOARTHRITIS

Parameter	Rheumatoid Arthritis	Osteoarthritis
Age	Young and middle-aged	Usually > 40 yr of age
Gender	Female more often than male	Same incidence
Weight	Weight loss	Usually overweight
Illness	Systemic manifestations	Local joint manifestations
Affected joints	PIPs, MCPs, MTPs, wrists, elbows, shoulders, knees, hips, cervical spine Usually bilateral	DIPs, first CMCs, thumbs, first MTPs knees, spine, hips; asymmetric, one or more joints
Effusions	Common	Uncommon
Nodules	Present	Heberden's nodes
Synovial fluid	Inflammatory	Noninflammatory
X-rays	Osteoporosis, narrowing, erosions	Osteophytes, subchondral cysts, sclerosis
Anemia	Common	Uncommon
Rheumatoid factor	Positive	Negative
Sedimentation rate	Elevated	Normal except in erosive osteoarthritis

From Lewis, S., Heitkemper, M., & Dirksen, S. (2000). *Medical-surgical nursing: Assessment and management of clinical problems* (5th ed., p. 1828). St. Louis, MO: Mosby. Reprinted with permission from Elsevier.

Etiology and Risk Factors

Osteoarthritis (OA) develops in men and women who are over 40 years of age; the incidence of OA tends to increase with age. Age is a significant risk factor for developing OA. While men and women are equally affected by OA in numbers, women appear to be more severely affected by the pathophysiological changes that occur (McCance & Mourad, 2000).

There are two forms of OA: primary idiopathic and secondary. The primary form of OA has no known risk factors. The secondary form of OA has identifiable risk factors that add stress to the joints, including but not limited to: trauma, congenital dislocations, occupational hazards, and sports. The primary form of OA is more common. The pathophysiology is the same in both forms of OA.

Pathophysiology

The pathophysiological changes associated with OA come about as a result of the erosion of the articular cartilage (McCance & Mourad, 2000). While the exact cause of the onset of OA is unknown, it is believed that the articular cartilage probably begins to break down as a result of enzyme activity. The articular cartilage is usually smooth, easing the movement of the bone ends as they come together within the joint. However, in OA the articular cartilage loses this smooth surface, gradually becoming discolored with cracks and roughened areas appearing in the surface of the cartilage. The cartilage over time thins out and erodes away from the surface of the bone, eventually leaving the bone ends to move upon each other unprotected by the cartilage. The underlying bone becomes sclerotic and begins to form new bony outgrowths called osteophytes. These osteophytes can break off within the joint cavity, causing irritation and inflammation to develop within the joint. These broken and loose pieces of bone are called joint mice; they can be seen on x-ray. The osteophytes continue to grow and lead to enlarged, deformed joints that eventually begin to lose function.

Clinical Manifestations

OA is not a systemic disease like RA, so there will be no systemic signs or symptoms. OA is also confined to the joints, which is another important difference between RA and OA. The signs and symptoms related to OA are joint manifestations. The joints are affected asymmetrically. The joints most commonly affected by OA are the weight-bearing joints of hips, knees and spine. The finger joints are frequently involved as well. Heberden's nodes and Bouchard's nodes are bony overgrowth nodules that develop in the finger joints (see Figure 12–3). These nodes can be swollen, red, and tender when inflammation is present (Bush, 2000).

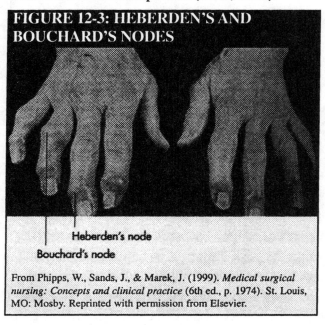

FIGURE 12-3: HEBERDEN'S AND BOUCHARD'S NODES

Heberden's node
Bouchard's node

From Phipps, W., Sands, J., & Marek, J. (1999). *Medical surgical nursing: Concepts and clinical practice* (6th ed., p. 1974). St. Louis, MO: Mosby. Reprinted with permission from Elsevier.

The patient will experience pain in one or more joints, especially upon weight-bearing and movement. The pain is relieved with rest. The joints may be stiff and enlarged. The stiffness usually occurs in the morning after getting out of bed but is transient, lasting less than 30 minutes. The range of motion in the joints becomes limited.

Crepitus, a grating sound, may be heard in the joint with movement (Pigg, 2000).

Diagnosis

The diagnosis of OA is difficult to make, as there are no laboratory studies indicative of OA and x-rays may not reveal joint changes until later in the disease. Diagnosis will be made based upon the patient's history and clinical manifestations.

Medical Management

There is no cure for OA. The treatment of OA is based upon the signs and symptoms that the patient is exhibiting. If the patient is overweight, a weight reduction diet will be suggested to decrease the stress on the weight-bearing joints. The patient may find the application of heat beneficial. Splints and braces may serve to immobilize and rest a painful joint. Assistive ambulatory devices, such as a walker, may help the patient bear weight on a painful joint by relieving some of the stress.

Pharmacological therapy will be used to help relieve the joint pain. Aspirin is no longer used in the treatment of OA. The drug of choice is acetaminophen, up to 1 gram four times a day (Bush, 2000). If acetaminophen is not effective, then NSAIDs will be added to the drug regimen. Corticosteroid injections may be used as necessary to treat individual joints that are acutely painful.

Surgical intervention becomes an option when the pain can no longer be controlled and the patient has lost function in the joint. Viscosupplementation is a new treatment for OA of the knee. It involves a series of intra-articular injections of hyaluronic acid into the knee to act as a lubricant within the joint. When effective, the pain can be relieved for up to 6 months (Pigg, 2000). Total joint replacement is also an option for those patients who have reached end-stage disease.

Nursing Care

The nursing care for a patient with OA is similar to that of a patient with RA in that the nurse's goal is to relieve pain and preserve joint mobility as long as possible. Patients are rarely hospitalized except when they are having surgery to replace the joint. Most of the patient contact will be in ambulatory clinics. The nurse should assess the patient's knowledge of the disease and treatment. Patient education on how to safely use adaptive devices, apply heat, and relieve stress on joints is important. The nurse should review the pharmacological therapy with the patient, including dosage and side effects.

Patients with OA are the most likely candidates for total joint replacement. The reader is referred to Chapter 14 for care of the patient undergoing a total joint replacement.

GOUT

Gout is an arthritis that is characterized by intermittent episodes of acute attacks caused by elevated serum uric acid levels (Lamb & Cummings, 2000). During the acute attacks of gouty arthritis, urate crystals cause joint inflammation. Gout can also be chronic in nature.

Etiology and Risk Factors

Gout can be either primary or secondary (acquired). Primary gout is an hereditary disorder of purine metabolism. There is an overproduction or decreased urinary excretion of uric acid, leading to elevated serum uric acid levels. Primary gout can also be caused by excessive dieting or eating foods high in purines (organ meats). Secondary, or acquired, gout is caused by medications that lead to uric acid retention or by other physical disorders that can lead to hyperuricemia (e.g., alcoholism, malignancies, renal disorders, diabetes, etc.). Middle-aged males are most likely to be affected by primary gout. Thiazide diuretics are an example of a commonly prescribed medication that can lead to secondary gout.

Pathophysiology

Hyperuricemia (elevated uric acid levels) can lead to the deposit of urate crystals in joints. The urate crystals initiate an inflammatory response within the joints, causing the joints to become painful, reddened, and warm to touch (Pigg, 2000). Over time, the urate crystals can accumulate in joint deposits that are called tophi.

Clinical Manifestations

Gout can be acute or chronic. Usually the initial onset of gout is sudden, with the patient complaining of acute discomfort in one or more joints (Lamb & Cummings, 2000). The great toe is most commonly affected by gout. A joint that is affected by an acute attack of gout is hot, swollen, and red. The pain can be severe with the patient unable to tolerate touch or move the joint. Besides the great toe, other joints that are affected by attacks of gout include the elbows, knees, wrists, and ankles. The patient may develop an elevated temperature and experience chills. The acute attack will eventually run its course in approximately 3–10 days, whether or not the patient seeks treatment. Chronic gout develops as a result of the urate crystal deposits (tophi) eventually leading to joint deformity. Tophi generally develop about 10 years after the initial diagnosis of gout (Pigg, 2000). The patient may also develop kidney stones as a result of the hyperuricemia (Lamb & Cummings, 2000).

Diagnosis

The diagnosis of gout is made based upon the clinical manifestations and laboratory findings. The patient will have a high serum uric acid level. Since gout is an inflammatory process, the patient may have an elevated white blood cell count and elevated sedimentation rate. X-rays may show the presence of tophi in the joints. Synovial fluid aspirations will demonstrate the presence of urate crystals.

Medical Management

The initial management of gout is accomplished with medications. During an acute attack of gout, a nonsteroidal anti-inflammatory (NSAID) may be prescribed. Colchicine, which reduces inflammation, may also be used during acute attacks. Colchicine may be administered orally or parenterally, usually until the pain decreases or the patient develops diarrhea. With colchicine, the pain usually begins to decrease within 48 hours (Lamb & Cummings, 2000). Corticosteroids may also be prescribed during the acute phase if colchicines and NSAIDs are not effective (Bush, 2000). Analgesics may also be prescribed for pain relief.

For prolonged treatment, a uricosuric agent such as probenecid (Benemid), which increases uric acid excretion, will be administered. Allopurinol (Zyloprim®), which blocks uric acid formation, is another drug that may be prescribed. Allopurinol has the potentially serious side effect of bone marrow depression that can limit its usefulness (Pigg, 2000). The prognosis for gout is good with the appropriate drug therapy.

Nursing Care

During the acute phase of gout, the primary nursing goal is to provide pain relief. The nurse must remember that the pain can be very acute — even the touch of clothing on the joint may be more than the patient can tolerate. The joint may need immobilization to decrease pain. The application of cold therapy may also provide some relief. The nurse should administer analgesics as necessary.

Patient education is also important. The nurse should instruct the patient to avoid alcohol and foods high in purines. Foods that are high in purines include organ meats and shellfish. Dietary restrictions are usually not difficult to follow and may not even be necessary if the drug therapy is effective. Reduction of weight, if the patient is obese, is also desirable to decrease strain on the joints. To avoid the development of kidney stones, the patient should also be instructed to increase fluid intake to 2000–3000 ml per day.

SUMMARY

Arthritis is a common chronic disease in the United States, with rheumatoid arthritis and osteoarthritis being two of the most common forms of the disease. Rheumatoid arthritis is an autoimmune, systemic, inflammatory disease, while osteoarthritis is essentially a degenerative disorder

that attacks individual joints. Gout is another form of arthritis caused by excessive uric acid that leads to inflammation of the joints. All of these forms of arthritis result in painful joints that can lead to disability. It is important that the nurse understand the basic pathophysiological differences between rheumatoid arthritis, osteoarthritis, and gout, as these differences have a bearing on the medical treatment and nursing care that will be provided. With adequate knowledge of these arthritic diseases, the nurse can effectively assist the patient in relieving pain and preserving joint function.

EXAM QUESTIONS

CHAPTER 12
Questions 80-84

80. Typical rheumatoid arthritis is

    a. associated with aging.

    b. localized to individual joints.

    c. bilaterally symmetrical in joint involve-
       ment.

    d. confined to weight-bearing joints only.

81. The pathophysiological changes related to
    rheumatoid arthritis can best be described as

    a. related to a degenerative process.

    b. related to an inflammatory process.

    c. a loss of articular cartilage due to structural
       wear.

    d. an infectious process affecting connective
       tissue.

82. The nurse caring for a patient who has
    rheumatoid arthritis should

    a. teach the patient to place joints in a flexed
       position to decrease pain.

    b. apply cold therapy to inflamed joints for
       20 minute intervals.

    c. place pillows under the patient's knees
       when resting to relieve strain.

    d. limit range-of-motion exercises to unin-
       volved joints.

83. One risk factor for osteoarthritis is

    a. joint trauma.

    b. large frame skeleton.

    c. male gender.

    d. low calcium intake.

84. Characteristic signs and symptoms of
    osteoarthritis are

    a. fatigue and malaise.

    b. pain unrelieved by rest.

    c. low grade fever.

    d. presence of Herberden's nodes.

CHAPTER 13

CARE OF PATIENTS WITH OSTEOPOROSIS

CHAPTER OBJECTIVE

After completing this chapter, the reader will be able to describe the nursing care of patients who have osteoporosis. In addition, health promotion activities that can help prevent the development of osteoporosis will be discussed.

LEARNING OBJECTIVES

After studying this chapter, the reader will be able to

1. identify the risk factors for the development of osteoporosis.

2. indicate the etiology and pathophysiology of osteoporosis.

3. specify the clinical manifestations of osteoporosis.

4. select the medical management and nursing care of patients with osteoporosis.

5. indicate health promotion activities to prevent the development of osteoporosis.

OVERVIEW

Osteoporosis is a metabolic bone disease that results in decreased bone density. It is the most common metabolic bone disease, with approximately 50% of all women developing osteoporosis at some point in their lives (McCance & Mourad, 2000). While osteoporosis is most common in women, especially post-menopausal white women, it also can occur in males. It is estimated that about 25 to 35 million people in the United States have osteoporosis (Ruda, 2000b). As the population of the United States continues to age, the incidence of osteoporosis will continue to increase. Osteoporosis is a leading cause of bone fractures in the elderly. This chapter addresses the nursing care of a patient with osteoporosis.

ETIOLOGY OF OSTEOPOROSIS

There are essentially two types of osteoporosis: primary and secondary. Primary osteoporosis is not associated with any underlying pathological condition, while secondary osteoporosis has an identifiable cause (Marek, 1999a). Osteoporosis can also be classified as generalized or regional, with the regional form of osteoporosis developing from a known cause and confined to a specific area of the skeleton (McCance & Mourad, 2000). Primary or generalized osteoporosis is the most common form of osteoporosis, and it usually involved large portions of the skeleton.

While the exact cause of primary osteoporosis is unknown, there are several risk factors associated with the development of the disease. Being female, thin, small in bone structure, white, and post-menopausal are some of the most significant risk factors (Ruda, 2000b). The loss of estrogen in menopause appears to be a factor in osteoporosis. Lack of calcium intake is also a factor in the development of osteoporosis. Excessive smoking and alcohol ingestion have also been identified as potential risk factors. Having a sedentary lifestyle can also increase the rate of bone loss (McCance & Mourad, 2000). It has been estimated that 60–80% of the risk that a woman will develop osteoporosis is inherited (Roberts & Lappe, 2001). Risk factors for osteoporosis are listed in Table 13–1.

TABLE 13–1: RISK FACTORS FOR PRIMARY OSTEOPOROSIS

Female gender

Slender build, small bone structure

Fair skinned

Caucasian

Familial history of osteoporosis

Post-menopausal (including surgically induced)

Calcium deficient diet

Lack of weight-bearing exercise

Smoking

Excessive alcohol intake

Source: Adapted from Lewis, Heitkemper, Dirksen. (2000). Medical surgical nursing: Assessment and management of clinical problems (5th ed.), St.Louis: Mosby.

Secondary osteoporosis is caused by an identifiable, underlying pathological condition. Certain chronic health conditions can predispose the individual to osteoporosis. Sometimes the long-term use of medications to treat other chronic health conditions can lead to the development of osteoporosis. For example, the long-term use of corticosteroids causes loss of bone mass (McCance & Mourad, 2000). Prolonged immobilization is another common cause of osteoporosis. Some examples of the most common risk factors that can lead to the development of secondary osteoporosis are listed in Table 13–2. Treatment of secondary osteoporosis is directed toward removing the underlying cause of bone loss (Marek, 1999a).

TABLE 13–2: EXAMPLES OF RISK FACTORS FOR SECONDARY OSTEOPOROSIS

Endocrine Disorders

Cushing syndrome

Hyperparathyroidism

Hyperthyroidism

Long-term drug use

Corticosteroid therapy

Thyroid replacement therapy

Antiseizure drugs

Loop diuretics (ex., furosemide)

Lithium

Heparin

Prolonged immobilization/Disuse

Chronic illness

Rheumatoid arthritis

Liver cirrhosis

Anorexia nervosa

Malabsorption

Kidney disease

Diabetes mellitus

Multiple myeloma

Source: Adapted from Phipps, Sanders, & Marek. (1999). Medical surgical nursing: concepts & clinical practice. St.Louis: Mosby.

PATHOPHYSIOLOGY

Regardless of the cause of osteoporosis, the pathophysiological process leading to loss of bone mass is the same. There is a disruption in the bone resorption and bone formation processes, which are normally carefully regulated and balanced. In osteoporosis, this process becomes unbalanced, with bone being resorbed at a rate faster than it can be formed. A decrease in bone density occurs, leading to the development of fragile bone that can no longer provide adequate structural support to the skeleton. The bone tissue that remains is normal from a histological and biochemical standpoint, there is just not enough of it (McCance & Mourad,

2000). While bone loss occurs throughout the skeleton, the most common sites for osteoporosis to develop are the wrists, hips and spine (Ruda, 2000b).

Bone loss that is age-related begins around the age of 40, with women losing more bone than men. The bone remodeling process in adults, consisting of bone resorption and formation, typically takes about 4 months for one cycle to be completed. In individuals with osteoporosis, the cycle can take almost 2 years to complete (Marek, 1999a).

CLINICAL MANIFESTATIONS

Many individuals develop osteoporosis without being aware of it, due to the silent nature of the disorder and the lack of symptoms. Frequently, it is the sudden occurrence of a bone fracture that leads to the diagnosis of osteoporosis (Roberts & Lappe, 2001).

When symptoms do occur, however, the most common manifestations of osteoporosis are pain and deformity. One of the most common sites for pain to develop is in the back when vertebrae collapse, resulting in a compression fracture of the vertebrae. The thoracic area is a common site of vertebral fractures. Kyphosis (dowager's hump) and loss of height are indications of collapsing vertebrae (Ruda, 2000b). Other common fracture sites include the long bones, radius, ribs, and femoral neck (McCance & Mourad, 2000).

It is important to remember that with osteoporosis, the bone can fracture with only minimal stress. It is estimated that close to 65,000 women die annually as a result of hip fractures and that approximately 50% of the individuals who have osteoporosis and suffer a fracture will never regain the ability to walk. The financial costs associated with osteoporosis are believed to be more than $13 billion in the United States (McCance & Mourad, 2000).

DIAGNOSING OSTEOPOROSIS

Osteoporosis cannot be diagnosed by x-ray until there has been a loss of more than 25–40% of the bone's calcium. Serum levels of phosphorus, calcium, and alkaline phosphatase may be evaluated, but they are usually within normal ranges (Ruda, 2000b). Laboratory tests and x-rays may also be conducted to rule out other medical disorders (Liddel, 2000).

One of the most common methods of determining bone density is through the measurement of bone mineral density (BMD). BMD measures bone mass and can be used to help predict individuals who are at a high risk for fracture. Individuals who have been diagnosed with osteoporosis should undergo measurement of their BMD every 1–2 years to monitor treatment response (Marek, 2000a). There are a variety of methods used to measure bone mineral density. One of the most common is dual x-ray absorptiometry (DXA), which can be used to determine the bone density of the hip, spine, and forearm with accuracy. DXA is the preferred test for measuring bone density because of the accuracy of the test (Lundon, 2000). One of the newer methods is the quantitative ultrasound (QUS) that measures bone density of the heel. The QUS is portable and less expensive than the DXA, and it is also sensitive enough to predict the risk for fracture (Marek, 1999a).

MEDICAL MANAGEMENT

The medical management of osteoporosis emphasizes weight-bearing exercise, adequate nutrition, calcium supplements, and pharmacological therapy. Daily weight-bearing exercise helps to maintain bone mass as well as muscle strength, coordination, and balance, thus decreasing the likelihood of falls and fractures. Walking is an ideal form of exercise as it promotes weight-bearing without undue stress on bones (Ruda, 2000b).

A diet that is rich in calcium and vitamin D is also important in the treatment of osteoporosis. Foods that are high in calcium are encouraged in the patient's diet. See Table 13–3 for a list of foods that are rich in calcium. Calcium supplements are prescribed to ensure an adequate intake of calcium. The goal for calcium intake is 1200–1500mg/daily (Liddel, 2000c).

TABLE 13–3: CALCIUM RICH FOODS
Dairy products (milk, cheese, ice cream, yogurt, etc.)
Broccoli
Spinach and other leafy greens
Salmon
Shrimps

Pharmacological therapy for the treatment of osteoporosis includes hormone replacement therapy (HRT). Other medications that may be prescribed include calcitonin, biphosphonates (Lundon, 2000), and estrogen receptor modulators (Ruda, 2000b).

HRT, consisting of estrogen, is prescribed for post-menopausal women to prevent the development of osteoporosis. The estrogen is believed to inhibit bone loss by decreasing bone resorption. Estrogen is combined with progesterone to decrease the risk of endometrial cancer. Other risks of estrogen therapy include an increased risk of breast cancer. Recent research in the Women's Health Initiative indicated that combination HRT, especially long-term HRT, may carry risks that exceed the benefits (Turkoski, 2002). Each woman must consider the risks and benefits of HRT when making the decision of whether or not to begin HRT. It is essential that women who elect to take HRT conduct monthly breast self-examination and have an annual pelvic examination with Pap smear (Liddel, 2000c). The greatest benefit of estrogen therapy appears to occur during the first 10 years after the onset of menopause (Ruda, 2000b).

Calcitonin is administered either intramuscularly, subcutaneously, or by nasal spray. Calcitonin is effective because it decreases the rate of bone loss through the inhibition of osteoclastic activity. Side effects of calcitonin therapy include nasal irritation (with use of nasal spray), nausea, and flushing. Teaching the patient to alternate nostrils when using the nasal spray will decrease the incidence of nasal irritation (Ruda, 2000b).

Biphosphonates are another classification of drugs used to treat osteoporosis. Biphosphonates act by inhibiting the resorption of bone and increasing bone mass. Alendronate (Fosamax®) is one of the most commonly prescribed biphosphonates; it appears to be particularly effective in reducing the incidence of fractures (Lundon, 2000).

Alendronate is known to cause gastrointestinal side effects such as nausea, heartburn, flatulence, constipation, or diarrhea (Liddel, 2000c). To increase absorption of the medication, the patient should be taught to take alendronate with a glass of water on an empty stomach first thing in the morning. The patient should then refrain from any eating or drinking any food or fluids for approximately 30 minutes after taking the medication. To decrease gastrointestinal side effects, the patient should also remain upright for at least 30 minutes after taking the medication (Ruda, 2000b).

Estrogen receptor modulators are another form of drug recently used in the treatment of osteoporosis (Ruda, 2000b). Estrogen receptor modulators have the same action as estrogen without the potential side effects of breast or endometrial cancer. Raloxifene (Evista®) is an example of an estrogen receptor modulator.

NURSING CARE

Health promotion and patient teaching are important aspects of the nurse's role when caring for patients who are at risk for osteoporosis. Health promotion activities that are implemented early enough can prevent or delay the development of osteoporosis, preserve function, and decrease the risk for fractures.

Health promotion activities should begin at an early age, especially in young women. It is important, however, to raise male awareness about the fact that men can develop osteoporosis, and in fact, have a greater chance of experiencing a hip fracture from osteoporosis than they do developing prostate cancer (Geier, 2001). Many men, and women, consider osteoporosis to be solely a women's disease. An awareness of the risk factors for osteoporosis is essential so that young individuals can make appropriate life style choices that will help increase and preserve bone mass. Instruction in how to achieve a balanced diet with an adequate intake of vitamin D and calcium rich foods is a key component of health promotion. Calcium supplements are appropriate for those who cannot achieve a satisfactory calcium intake (1200–1500 mg/day) through diet alone. Individuals should also be instructed to avoid certain activities that can inhibit calcium absorption and increase bone loss — smoking, alcohol use, and caffeinated beverages. The benefits of an active lifestyle in preventing osteoporosis are significant. Weight-bearing activities that also promote muscle activity help increase bone formation and improve coordination and muscle strength.

As women age and become post-menopausal, they should be educated about the benefits and risks of HRT so that they can make an informed decision about the use of such therapy to prevent osteoporosis. In addition, the risk of fractures is increased with aging and bone density loss. Individuals should be encouraged to participate in screening activities to determine their BMD. The nurse should incorporate safety factors related to developing a safe home environment and preventing falls into patient teaching plans. It is important to teach individuals about correct body mechanics as spontaneous bone fractures, especially in the thoracic vertebral areas, can easily occur as a result of falls, sud-

den movements, bending, twisting, or straining activities when osteoporosis is present.

Another aspect of nursing care that should be considered is the patient's psychosocial needs (Lundon, 2000). Osteoporosis often leads to deformity such as kyphosis, as the vertebrae collapse upon themselves. The patient suffers a loss of height, pain, and a potential loss of function. The back rounds and the abdomen develops a protruding appearance. Clothing fits poorly. These changes in appearance and function are permanent and can cause an alteration in body image and self-esteem. The patient may become depressed. The nurse should be sensitive to these potential psychosocial issues and encourage the patient to verbalize feelings and concerns.

SUMMARY

Osteoporosis is currently the most common metabolic bone disorder present in the United States, with the incidence of osteoporosis predicted to increase as the population continues to age. While osteoporosis is most common in women, it is important to remember that men can also develop osteoporosis. The consequences of osteoporosis can be debilitating. Osteoporosis can be prevented, or the onset delayed, by implementing the appropriate life style modifications. The earlier these modifications are made, the more likely that the individual will be able to preserve bone mass. The nurse plays a key role in teaching the patient health promotion activities to prevent the development of osteoporosis.

CASE STUDY

Mrs. J.G. is a 50 year-old woman who is approaching menopause. She has come into the physician's office for her annual physical examination. She is slender in build and has fair skin. During the health history, she tells you she smokes one pack of cigarettes a day but that she is trying to *quit. Mrs. J.G. also mentions that her job as an executive secretary is very sedentary and she does not exercise regularly. She tells you that she is concerned about developing osteoporosis. Her elderly mother developed osteoporosis and suffered a fractured hip from a fall. Mrs. J.G. tells you she does not want to experience the same health problems her mother has experienced.*

Answer the following case study questions, writing your responses on a separate sheet of paper. Compare your responses to the answers that are located at the end of the chapter.

1. What are the risk factors associated with osteoporosis?

2. Mrs. J. G. wants to know what she can do to lessen the likelihood that she will develop osteoporosis. What do you tell her?

3. What are some of the calcium-rich foods that Mrs. J.G. can incorporate into her diet?

4. Mrs. J.G. tells you that she enjoys swimming and wants to know if it is an effective exercise for preventing the development of osteoporosis. What information can you give her about activity and exercise related to preventing osteoporosis?

5. The doctor prescribes alendronate (Fosamax®) for Mrs. J.G. You are providing Mrs. J.G. with instructions on how to correctly take the medication. What information should you include in your teaching session?

Answers to Case Study

1. Risk factors for osteoporosis include being female, post-menopausal, slight of build, and fair-skinned. Caucasian women have a higher incidence of osteoporosis. Individuals with a family history of osteoporosis have a higher risk as well. Additional risk factors include a calcium-deficient diet, lack of weight-bearing exercise, smoking, and excessive alcohol intake.

2. Mrs. J.G. would benefit from increasing the amount of weight-bearing exercise in her life and stopping smoking. Increasing the amount of calcium and vitamin D in her diet would also be beneficial, as would taking a calcium supplement. She would benefit from bone density testing to measure her current bone mass and her likelihood for developing osteoporosis.

3. Some of the calcium-rich foods that Mrs. J. G. can incorporate into her diet includes dairy products (milk, cheese, ice cream, yogurt, etc.), broccoli, spinach, and other leafy greens. Some fish, such as salmon and shrimp, is also high in calcium.

4. While swimming has many benefits, it is not a weight-bearing exercise and is not effective for preventing osteoporosis. Weight-bearing exercises, such as walking, help promote muscle activity, increase bone formation, and improve coordination and muscle strength. Mrs. J.G. should be encouraged to engage in weight-bearing exercise

5. Alendronate (Fosamax®) is a biphosphonate. Fosamax® works by inhibiting the resorption of the bone and increasing bone mass. Common side effects include nausea, heartburn, flatulence, constipation, and diarrhea. Mrs. J. G. should be instructed to take the medication on an empty stomach with a full glass of water to promote absorption of the drug. Mrs. J.G. should then avoid eating and drinking for 30 minutes after taking the medication. She should also remain upright after taking the medication.

EXAM QUESTIONS

CHAPTER 13
Questions 85-90

85. One risk factor for osteoporosis is

    a. obesity.

    b. small bone structure.

    c. being a caucasian male.

    d. occasional alcohol intake.

86. The pathological process that leads to osteo-porosis is

    a. the development of an infection within the bone.

    b. a lack of blood flow to the bone.

    c. disruption in the balance between bone resorption and formation.

    d. an inability to absorb calcium into the bone.

87. Clinical manifestations of osteoporosis may include

    a. development of deformities.

    b. swollen joints.

    c. feeling of malaise.

    d. muscle contractures.

88. A health promotion activity that is important in the prevention of osteoporosis is

    a. encouraging the patient to participate in range of motion exercises daily.

    b. avoiding the use of non-steroidal anti-inflammatory drugs.

    c. increasing the intake of calcium to 1200–1500 mg/day.

    d. getting at least 8 hours of sleep every night.

89. Raloxifene (Evista®) is an example of

    a. an estrogen receptor modulator.

    b. hormone replacement therapy.

    c. a biphosphonate.

    d. a calcium supplement.

90. A patient who has just been started on Fosamax® (alendronate) for the treatment of osteoporosis should be told to

    a. always take Fosamax® with food.

    b. have calcium blood levels monitored monthly.

    c. take Fosamax® at bedtime.

    d. sit or stand upright for 30 minutes after taking Fosamax®.

CHAPTER 14

CARE OF PATIENTS WITH A TOTAL JOINT REPLACEMENT

CHAPTER OBJECTIVE

After completing this chapter, the reader will be able to describe the medical management and nursing care of patients who have experienced a total joint replacement.

LEARNING OBJECTIVES

After studying this chapter, the reader will be able to

1. identify the conditions that will most likely cause a patient to have a total joint replacement.

2. specify the preoperative nursing care for a patient who is undergoing a total joint replacement.

3. indicate the postoperative nursing care for a patient who has had a total joint replacement of the hip or knee.

4. identify the potential complications related to a total joint replacement.

5. select the principles of rehabilitation for the patient who has experienced a total joint replacement.

OVERVIEW

Total joint replacement, or arthroplasty, is indicated for patients who are suffering from severe joint pain or loss of function. Total joint replacement surgery is one of the most common forms of orthopedic surgery performed on the elderly. Recent advances in surgical technique and prosthetic design have greatly improved the outcomes for these surgeries (Bush, 2000). Many patients who suffer from degenerative joint disease have experienced a decrease in pain and an increase in functional ability as a result of joint replacement surgery.

Total joint replacement surgery is indicated when other treatment regimens have not been successful, so the patient is losing functional ability and experiencing serious pain (Roberts & Lappe, 2001). Some of the conditions that may cause degeneration of a joint and lead to the need for replacement surgery are rheumatoid arthritis, degenerative joint disease (osteoarthritis), femoral neck fractures that result in avascular necrosis, and trauma. Congenital deformities may be an indication for a joint replacement (Liddel, 2000c).

Total joint replacement prostheses may be made of metal, high-density polyethylene, ceramic, or other synthetic materials (Marek, 1999b). The most common joint replacements are for the hips and knees. Finger joints are also commonly replaced. Other joints that can be replaced, but are more complex, include the ankle, shoulder, elbow, and wrist (Liddel, 2000c). See Figure 14–1 to see an illustration of hip and knee replacement prostheses.

A prosthesis that is cemented in with a bone bonding agent may be used, or else a non-cemented, ingrowth prosthesis is used. Cemented prostheses

FIGURE 4-1: HIP AND KNEE REPLACEMENT PROSTHESES

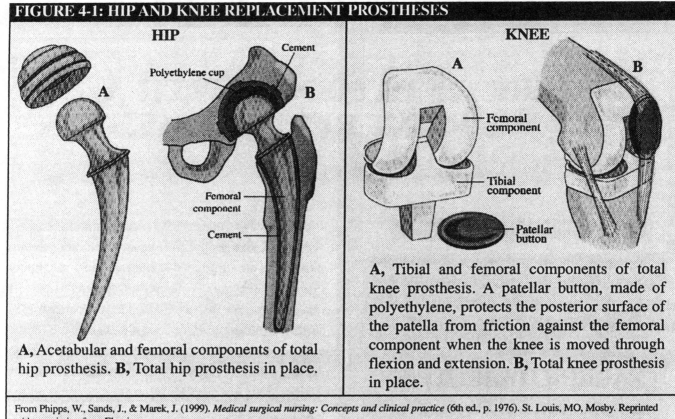

A, Acetabular and femoral components of total hip prosthesis. **B,** Total hip prosthesis in place.

A, Tibial and femoral components of total knee prosthesis. A patellar button, made of polyethylene, protects the posterior surface of the patella from friction against the femoral component when the knee is moved through flexion and extension. **B,** Total knee prosthesis in place.

From Phipps, W., Sands, J., & Marek, J. (1999). *Medical surgical nursing: Concepts and clinical practice* (6th ed., p. 1976). St. Louis, MO, Mosby. Reprinted with permission from Elsevier.

provide the advantage of an immediate fixation of the device. However, over time the cement may fail and lead to loosening of the prosthesis. If the prosthesis becomes loose, another surgery is required to revise and replace the joint. Porous, ingrowth prostheses allow bone to grow in and around the prosthesis to eventually secure it to the bone. This prosthesis will not loosen and it is believed to last longer, but it takes some time for the bone to grow into the prosthesis and stabilize the joint. Currently more ingrowth prostheses are being inserted than those which require cement (Liddel, 2000c). Which prosthesis the surgeon uses will depend on a number of factors — the age of the patient, weight, activity, and the physical condition and blood supply of the remaining bone (Marek, 1999b).

PREOPERATIVE NURSING CARE FOR JOINT REPLACEMENT SURGERY

Most joint replacement surgeries are elective surgeries, so the patient has time to prepare for the surgical experience. The goal of the preoperative period is to have the patient in the best health possible to facilitate a full recovery following surgery. Preoperatively, the patient will be assessed for any co-existing health problems to be sure that these physical conditions are being adequately controlled. Special attention will be paid to the patient's cardiovascular, respiratory, and renal status. The weight of the person will also be taken into consideration. Obese individuals may not be candidates for total joint replacement surgery until weight loss has occurred, due to the potential for postoperative complications and stressors placed on the prosthesis from the extra weight (Liddel, 2000c).

Patient education is important prior to surgery in order to prepare the patient for the postoperative period. The patient will be instructed about the procedure, the potential complications following surgery, expectations for ambulation, available methods of pain control, and the nursing care that will be provided following surgery. The patient is given time to ask any questions he or she may have about the procedure. Since many patients will be admitted to the hospital the day of the procedure, the patient teaching that occurs prior to this time as an outpatient is important to preparing the patient adequately. Videos, written instructions, and brochures may all be useful methods of conveying information.

Prior to admission to the hospital for surgery, the patient should be encouraged to stop smoking to improve respiratory functioning. The patient should be assessed for the presence of any infection. Surgery will be postponed for any patient who has an infection. Infection, if present, can predispose the patient to infection at the prosthesis site and increase the potential for developing osteomyelitis. Every precaution is taken to avoid infection. Prophylactic antibiotics probably will be administered preoperatively. Skin preparation at the operative site will begin 1 to 2 days prior to surgery.

It is also beneficial for the patient to maintain his or her level of functional ability prior to surgery, as this may shorten the postoperative rehabilitation time (Ditmyer, Topp, & Pifer, 2002). The patient will also be instructed in leg exercises and muscle strengthening exercises to aid in ambulation following surgery. The patient may be fitted with assistive walking devices preoperatively.

Since blood loss during orthopedic surgery can be significant, patients may wish to participate in autologous donation of blood, which is the donation of their own blood to be reinfused into them at a later date during surgery. This prevents the need for the patient to receive blood from another individual. Another option for autologous blood transfusion is the use of a salvage and reinfusion blood device that can be used in surgery (Warner, 2001). Some surgeons prefer this method of autologous blood transfusion, which saves the patient from having to predonate blood for surgery.

Patients who are having a knee or hip joint replaced are at a particular risk for developing deep vein thrombosis (DVT) after surgery. DVT is one of the most common complications of total joint replacement surgery (Rice & Walsh, 2001). For this reason, patients will be given a dose of heparin or low-molecular-weight heparin as a prophylactic precaution. Patients who routinely take aspirin, steroids, anticoagulant therapy, or non-steroidal anti-inflammatory medications will be asked to stop these medications prior to surgery so as not to interfere with coagulation studies and wound healing. The steroids must be tapered off gradually prior to the surgery (Liddel, 2000).

The nurse will also want to address postoperative pain control with the patient prior to surgery. Patient-controlled analgesia is used. The patient should be instructed in how to use the pump and how to operate the delivery device to administer medication.

POSTOPERATIVE CARE FOR A PATIENT WITH A TOTAL HIP REPLACEMENT

Total hip replacement involves the replacement of the femoral head and the acetabulum, most frequently due to arthritis. Typically, the femoral head is replaced with a metal component and the acetabulum is replaced with a plastic component. Following surgery for a total hip replacement, the nurse's primary goals of care are to promote mobility, prevent dislocation of the prosthesis, monitor drainage from the wound, prevent DVT, and prevent infection. The general care of the patient with a total hip replacement is similar to the care of any postoperative patient.

Patients will usually begin ambulation 1–2 days after surgery. The orthopedic surgeon will prescribe specific weight-bearing requirements for the extremity. If the patient has received a cemented prosthesis, it is likely that weight-bearing will be prescribe as tolerated by the patient. If the patient has received an ingrowth prosthesis, weight-bearing will be limited until the prosthesis has been stabilized by the ingrowth of bone (Liddel, 2000c). The patient must wear secure, well-fitting walking shoes when ambulating. The patient will always transfer from the bed in the direction of the unaffected leg.

As the patient begins moving in bed and ambulating, it is important that extremes of joint movement be avoided to prevent dislocation of the prosthesis. For example, internal rotation of the hip and adduction is avoided, and the hip is never flexed past 90 degrees (Bush, 2000). When in bed the patient should have an abduction splint or pillow in place between the legs to prevent accidental adduction of the hip. The head of the bed is not elevated past 60 degrees to avoid hip flexion. The patient is usually not turned to the operative side (Marek, 1999b). When the patient is repositioned in the bed, he or she is encouraged to flex the non-operated leg to assist with movement and to use the overhead trapeze. The patient never pushes off with or flexes the operated leg.

When up, the patient will use toilet seat extenders to avoid hip flexion and high-seated chairs that are firm. The knees should be lower than the hip when the patient is sitting. If the patient requires a wheelchair, it must be able to recline to prevent hip flexion. The patient is cautioned not to bend over or cross the legs. Tub baths are not allowed. The patient will require assistive devices to put on socks or shoes. Occupational therapists and physical therapists will work with the patient to teach safe ambulation techniques and to teach the patient how to adapt the activities of daily living to the current activity restrictions. The patient will need to contin-

ue to implement hip precautions for about 4 months after the surgery (Liddel, 2000c).

Encouraging the patient with early ambulation and instructing the patient about hourly leg exercises will help prevent the development of DVT. In addition, the nurse administers prophylactic heparin therapy and encourages fluid intake. The nurse should also assess the patient's legs every 4 hours for signs of redness, swelling, or tenderness. Frequent neurovascular checks are performed to detect alterations in the affected extremity's circulation. Anti-embolic stockings are used to support venous return. DVT is the most common complication following hip surgery, so the nurse must be vigilant to prevent the development of clots.

Postoperatively, the patient will have a wound drain for 24–48 hours to prevent the development of a hematoma (Marek, 1999b). Drainage during the first 24 hours is expected to average about 500 mL. The drainage gradually decreases to less than 30 mL in 8 hours. The drain is removed within 48 hours if the drainage has decreased as anticipated.

One of the most serious complications that can occur in joint replacement surgery is the onset of an infection. Wound care is provided using strict asepsis. The wound site is inspected frequently for redness or drainage. Wound drains are removed as quickly as possible. Antibiotics are prophylactically administered postoperatively for 2–3 days to help prevent the development of an infection (Roberts & Lappe, 2001). In addition, whenever the patient requires any invasive procedures in the future, such as dental procedures, prophylactic antibiotics will be administered. If an infection develops, it can be difficult to heal and may result in the need to remove and replace the prosthesis. Functional ability may be lost with the revision.

POSTOPERATIVE CARE FOR A PATIENT WITH A TOTAL KNEE REPLACEMENT

Patients who are experiencing severe pain in the knee due to a degenerative process are candidates for a knee replacement. The joint replacement will provide the patient with a pain-free joint and returned functional ability. Postoperative care of the patient and postoperative complications are similar to those of the patient with a total hip replacement.

Immediately postoperatively, the knee is wrapped in a compression bandage to provide immobilization and keep the knee extended. Ice may be applied to decrease swelling and pain. Neurovascular checks must be performed hourly in the immediate postoperative period. A wound drain is inserted for the first 24 hours after surgery. The drain is removed after drainage decreases to less than 30 mL/hour (Liddel, 2000c). In contrast to immobilizing the knee during the immediate postoperative period, some orthopedic surgeons prefer to place the patient's knee in the continuous passive motion (CPM) device immediately following surgery to passively flex the knee.

After the compression bandage is removed, a knee immobilizer is applied to protect the joint whenever the patient is ambulating or not exercising the joint. Exercise is important to regaining function. The knee will be placed in the CPM device that passively flexes the knee to a pre-determined level of flexion (Marek, 1999b). The surgeon will prescribe the degrees of flexion and length of time the CPM device should be used (Kotch, 2001). The patient is encouraged to use the CPM device as much as possible while in bed; at the very least, the patient should use the device 6–8 hours a day (Roberts & Lappe, 2001). Use of the device helps control swelling, decrease pain, and increase function. The use of CPM may be contraindicated in some patients who are at risk for poor wound heal-ing. Proper positioning on the device is important. The nurse should ensure that the knee is centered on the device and that the leg is in a position of neutral rotation (Kotch, 2001).

Ambulation is usually started within 24 hours of surgery, beginning with transferring the patient from the bed to the chair. The patient does not need to worry about prosthesis dislocation with a knee replacement, as is necessary with a hip replacement. Weight-bearing will be determined by the physician. Range of motion and leg strengthening exercises are important for mobility and function. The patient is encouraged to continue these exercises at home after discharge to maintain muscle strength. The patient must be instructed in how to use the prescribed ambulatory devices (walker, crutches) safely (Roberts & Lappe, 2001).

REHABILITATION FOLLOWING TOTAL JOINT SURGERY

Discharge planning for the patient with total joint replacement surgery begins during the preoperative phase of care. Following surgery, most patients are hospitalized for about 4 days. Some patients may be discharged to an extended care facility where they will continue to receive physical therapy, but others will return to their home. Patients are likely to be discharged home if they can transfer themselves from the bed and are able to ambulate safely and independently (Roberts & Lappe, 2001). Teaching the patient how to perform personal care is essential.

Prior to discharge, the home environment must be assessed for ease of access and safety. Are there stairs to be negotiated? Are the doorways and hallways large enough to accommodate a walker? Are throw rugs on the floor or pieces of furniture positioned in a way that they are easy to trip over? Are there pets? Is the bathroom accessible? If the patient has had a hip replacement, is a toilet extender available? Who is available to assist the patient in the home? Family members? Will home health aides be necessary? The nurse can help the patient and family consider how home care will be accomplished. The nurse can also tell the patient about community resources that may be available to provide assistance.

The patient will gradually be able to resume activities. Driving is not allowed for at least six weeks. Low-impact exercises, such as walking, swimming, or golfing, can be enjoyed as the patient's strength continues to return. High-impact activities are not recommended, as they place added stress upon the prosthetic device. The patient may want to know when sexual activity can be resumed. Since many patients may be reluctant to address this issue, it is up to the nurse to do so. Typically, sexual intercourse can be resumed about 8 weeks following hip replacement surgery. It is important that the patient continue to maintain proper positioning for the joint and avoid extreme hip flexion and rotation, as well as adduction (Marek, 1999b).

Patients should know that the rehabilitation phase will take about 1 year following surgery and that functional ability will continue to improve beyond that time. It may be 3 years following surgery before the patient achieves maximum functional ability (Marek, 1999). The patient must understand the importance of continuing to do daily exercise throughout this time period to be able to reach maximum function. It is easy for the patient to become discouraged during this time period; social support is an essential component to the patient's success. With persistent attention to the rehabilitation process, most patients are again able to function pain free and resume activities that they had previously found too painful to attempt.

SUMMARY

Due to improved surgical techniques and resilient prosthetic devices, many patients have successfully had total joint replacement sur-gery to help them regain function and eliminate severe pain from their lives. The nurse plays an important role in preparing the patient for surgery and aggressively providing postoperative nursing care, with the primary goal of preventing complications and supporting the patient through the rehabilitation phase of recovery.

EXAM QUESTIONS

CHAPTER 14
Questions 91-95

91. The conditions most likely to cause a patient to need a total joint replacement is

    a. osteoporosis.

    b. osteomyelitis.

    c. osteoarthritis.

    d. osteomalacia.

92. The primary goal of the preoperative nursing care for a patient undergoing a total joint replacement is to

    a. help the patient understand the complexity of the surgery.

    b. ensure the patient's health status is at an optimum level.

    c. prepare the patient for a lengthy period of immobility.

    d. rest the affected joint prior to surgery.

93. Following a total joint replacement for the hip, the nurse tells the patient he will begin ambulating

    a. 1–2 days after surgery.

    b. as soon as the pain decreases.

    c. when weight-bearing is allowed.

    d. after he learns to use a walker.

94. A potentially serious complication following total joint replacement surgery is

    a. muscle spasms.

    b. allergy to the prosthesis.

    c. wound infection.

    d. development of osteomalacia.

95. The nurse who is teaching a patient how to make the home environment safe for ambulation following a total joint replacement should recommend

    a. eliminating all animals from the home.

    b. removing throw rugs from the floors.

    c. not carrying anything while walking.

    d. sitting at a table while preparing dinner.

CHAPTER 15

CARE OF THE PATIENT
WITH A BONE NEOPLASM

CHAPTER OBJECTIVE

After completing this chapter, the reader will be able to describe the medical management and nursing care of patients who have a bone neoplasm or tumor. In addition, the care of a patient who has an amputation is discussed.

LEARNING OBJECTIVES

After studying this chapter, the reader will be able to:

1. identify the differences between a benign and malignant bone neoplasm.

2. specify the clinical manifestations of a bone neoplasm.

3. indicate the medical management of a primary malignant bone neoplasm.

4. identify the nursing care of a patient who has a primary malignant bone neoplasm.

5. identify the nursing care of a patient who experiences an amputation.

OVERVIEW

Bone neoplasms, or tumors, may be benign or malignant. There are various types of neoplasms that affect bone and the soft tissues. Benign neoplasms are much more common than malignant bone neoplasms.

Malignant bone neoplasms may be primary or metastatic. Primary malignant bone neoplasms are relatively rare and account for less than 1% of deaths from cancer (Ruda, 2000b). Most bone malignancies are metastatic, originating most commonly in the breast, lungs, or ovaries. Table 15–1 identifies some of the classifications of benign and malignant musculoskeletal tumors.

This chapter will address the nursing care of patients who have a primary malignant bone neoplasm. Many of the individuals who develop a primary malignant bone neoplasm are children or young adults. While the combination therapy of radiation, chemotherapy, and advanced surgical treatment have increased the chances for survival, the diagnosis of bone cancer is still devastating to the patient and family. Some patients may even require an amputation in an attempt to remove the malignancy. The nurse has a major role in providing support to the patient and family during diagnosis, treatment, and rehabilitation.

BENIGN BONE NEOPLASMS

Benign bone neoplasms are much more common than malignant neoplasms. As with most other benign neoplasms, the tumors are slow-growing, well-defined, and non-invasive. They typically do not cause pain or other symptoms and may go undetected for some time. They are not fatal and most do not require treatment.

TABLE 15–1: CLASSIFICATION OF BENIGN AND MALIGNANT MUSCULOSKELETAL NEOPLASMS

	Benign Tumors	Malignant Tumors
Bone	Osteoma	Osteosarcoma
Skeletal Muscle	Rhabdomyoma	Rhabdomyosarcoma
Fibrous Tissue	Fibroma	Fibrosarcoma
Cartilage	Chondroma	Chondrosarcoma
Fatty Tissue	Lipoma	Liposarcoma

Source: Adapted from Bender, C., Yasko, J. & Strohl, R. (2000). Cancer. In S.M. Lewis, M.M. Heitkemper, & S.R. Dirksen, (Eds.), *Medical-surgical nursing: Assessment and management of clinical problems* (5th ed.). St. Louis: Mosby, Inc., pp. 269–322.

There are, however, some benign bone neoplasms that are more aggressive and invasive in their growth patterns. Giant cell tumors, also known as osteoclastomas, are aggressive tumors that invade surrounding tissues and cause destruction in the bone. They develop in the cancellous ends of the bone, most commonly in the proximal tibia, distal femur, and distal radius (Ruda, 2000b). They are painful and can eventually become malignant. They most commonly occur in young adults 20–40 years old (Roberts & Lappe, 2001). With these types of tumors, surgical removal is indicated. Following surgery, the likelihood of reoccurrence is 50%. Amputation of the extremity may ultimately be required to contain the disease. Chemotherapy has improved the patient's chances of survival (Ruda, 2000b).

PRIMARY MALIGNANT BONE NEOPLASMS

Primary malignant bone neoplasms are relatively rare, with an estimated 2500 new cases diagnosed yearly (Roberts & Lappe, 2001). The most commonly diagnosed primary malignant bone neoplasms include osteosarcoma and Ewing's sarcoma. The etiology of these malignancies is unknown. Environmental exposure to toxins is thought to play some role in the development of the tumors. Most of the primary malignant bone tumors are aggressive in their growth and destruction. They most commonly occur in children or young adults. This chapter will focus discussion on two of the most commonly diagnosed primary malignant bone tumors — osteosarcoma and Ewing's sarcoma.

Osteosarcoma

Osteosarcoma, also known as osteogenic sarcoma, is the most common primary malignancy of the bone. It is a highly malignant tumor and is frequently fatal. It is most common in young males between the ages of 10 and 25. It can also develop in older individuals who have a history of Paget's disease. Unfortunately, by the time most patients report their symptoms to a physician the disease has already metastasized to the lungs. This early metastasis accounts for the high number of fatalities associated with this cancer (Liddel, 2000c).

Clinical manifestations of osteosarcoma include localized pain, swelling, and, eventually, a loss of function. Sometimes the first notable indication of the tumor is a mild limp. The tumor is most likely to develop in the metaphysis of the long bones. The most common sites of tumor growth are the proximal humerus, proximal tibia, and distal femur. The pelvis is another potential site (Ruda, 2000b).

The diagnosis of osteosarcoma is made by MRI, CT scan, and bone biopsy. A chest x-ray will be taken to determine if metastasis to the lungs has occurred. Laboratory studies will probably demonstrate an elevation in the serum alkaline phosphatase and serum calcium levels due to bone destruction.

Medical management has made advances in recent years so that the 5–year survival rate of patients with osteosarcoma is now 60% (Ruda, 2000b). The treatment is aggressive, starting with chemotherapy to shrink the size of the tumor before surgery. At one point, amputation was the only treatment of choice. Today, many patients are candidates for limb-salvage procedures, in which the tumor and surrounding tissues are removed and a prosthetic device is inserted. Bone grafts or joint replacements may also be a part of the surgical treatment. Chemotherapy will be administered again following the surgical removal of the tumor to decrease the likelihood of metastasis.

In some cases, due to the size and location of the tumor, the patient is not a candidate for a limb-salvage procedure. Amputation of the extremity is the only other option. The amputation will extend well above the location of the tumor to ensure total removal of the primary tumor and surrounding tissues (Liddel, 2000c).

Ewing's Sarcoma

Ewing's sarcoma is another primary bone malignancy that occurs most commonly in young adult males. Ewing's sarcoma grows aggressively and develops within the medullary cavity of the long bones. The high incidence of fatalities associated with this malignancy is the result of lung metastasis.

The signs and symptoms of Ewing's sarcoma include localized pain and swelling. The patient is likely to experience fever and leukocytosis. The tumor may also become palpable. The disease is diagnosed through x-rays that demonstrate the bone destruction.

Treatment consists of surgical excision and potentially amputation. Radiation therapy has been proven effective in treatment and is used in conjunction with the surgical removal of the tumor and chemotherapy. The combined usage of radiation, surgery, and chemotherapy have led to a 5-year survival rate of 70% for these patients (Ruda, 2000b).

NURSING CARE OF THE PATIENT WITH A PRIMARY MALIGNANT BONE NEOPLASM

The primary goals of nursing care for the patient with a malignant bone neoplasm include providing pain relief, helping the patient develop coping strategies, educating the patient regarding the disease and prognosis, and avoiding complications. Since many of these patients will undergo surgery to remove the tumor, postoperative nursing care will be necessary.

Aggressive pain control is a primary focus of nursing care. Pharmacological and non-pharmacological methods of pain control are used. Opioids, delivered through patient-controlled analgesic pumps, are usually used to relieve postoperative pain. Non-pharmacological methods of pain control include relaxation techniques and imagery. These methods of pain control are used in conjunction with analgesics, not in place of the medication.

It is also important that the affected extremity be handled very carefully and gently to minimize pain. When moving the involved limb, the nurse should always support it above and below the location of the tumor area. Bone that has been weakened by a tumor is susceptible to pathological fractures. Splints may be applied to support the extremity. The patient is likely to need assistive devices to minimize weight-bearing on the extremity.

The majority of the patients who develop primary malignant bone neoplasms are young and accustomed to being healthy. The sudden diagnosis of an aggressive form of cancer is particularly devastating to the patient and family. In addition, the treatment for the cancer will probably require surgical alterations of the extremity, maybe even amputation, as well as aggressive treatment with radiation and chemotherapy. The patients and their families require significant support as they strive to cope with these changes in their lives. The nurse needs to be available to listen to the patient's fears and concerns. It is appropriate to refer the patient and family to counseling so that they will get the support they need during this time period.

The nurse will also want to help the patient cope with the changes in body image and self-esteem that may occur due to surgery and amputation. The patient has usually been very independent and in control of life until the diagnosis of cancer. The nurse should continue to encourage independence and participation in the activities of daily living as much as possible. The nurse helps the patient develop a realistic understanding of the medical condition and provides realistic reassurance as appropriate. The patient should be encouraged to participate in the planning of care as much as possible to regain a feeling of control and independence.

NURSING CARE OF THE PATIENT WHO HAS AN AMPUTATION

While the current, progressive treatment of primary bone cancers has decreased the reliance on amputation as the treatment of choice, it is still true that patients who have bone cancer may need to have a limb amputated to save their lives. As many patients who have an amputation will be hospitalized on an orthopedic unit, the orthopedic nurse must be familiar with the nursing care required of the patient who has had an amputation.

In most cases of amputation, the amputation is performed at the most distal point possible that will provide for successful healing, and the objective is to preserve as much of the limb as feasible. In the case of primary malignant bone cancer, the objective is slightly different. The surgeon's goal is to remove as much of the extremity as necessary to ensure that the primary tumor and any potential regional metastasis has been eliminated. Due to the location of the malignant tumor, usually near the knee, it is quite likely that the majority of lower limb amputations due to malignant bone tumors will be above the knee (AK).

Preoperatively, the nurse will evaluate the patient's health status so that the patient can be in the best possible condition to withstand the surgery and promote wound healing. As the patient's nutritional status is particularly important to supporting wound healing, the nurse will want to ensure that the patient's diet is well balanced and includes adequate protein and vitamins. The nurse should also assess the patient's understanding of the procedure and psychological coping with the impending loss of an extremity. The nurse should reassure the patient that grief over the loss of a limb is normal and suggest counseling to help the patient cope. Patients may also benefit from clergy support to help meet spiritual needs and cope with the impending loss.

Following surgery, the nurse's primary goals are to control pain, support wound healing, provide psychological support, and help prepare the patient for the rehabilitation period following the amputation.

Pain control is achieved by the administration of opioid analgesics. Muscle spasms may contribute to the patient's discomfort. Patients are likely to experience phantom limb sensation, where it feels as if the amputated limb is still present. The patient may feel as if the limb is tingling or itching. An aching sensation may be described. The patient needs reassurance that these feelings are normal and will eventually disappear, usually over a matter of months.

Depending upon the surgeon's preference, the residual limb may either have a cast dressing in place or a soft dressing wrapped on the limb. Patients who have AK amputations usually will have delayed prosthetic fitting after the wound has healed (Ruda, 2000b). While awaiting the fitting of the prosthetic device, it is important that the residual limb is properly wrapped and positioned. Careful wrapping of the limb will help shape it and make it easier to fit the prosthesis. During the early postoperative period, it is important that the residual limb remain properly wrapped to decrease edema. Edema can interfere with the fitting of the prosthesis. Figure 15–1 shows the proper way to wrap a residual limb with an AK amputation.

The residual limb should be positioned to avoid the development of a hip flexion contracture. If the patient develops a flexion contracture of the hip, it prevents the patient from being able to ambulate with a prosthesis. The residual limb should not be elevated on a pillow, and the patient should be taught not to sit for prolonged periods with the hips flexed. If the patient is able to tolerate the prone position, he should be encouraged to lie prone 3–4 times a day for about 30 minutes each time so that the hip is extended. This will decrease the likelihood of a hip flexion contracture.

FIGURE 15-1: METHODS FOR BANDAGING AMPUTATION STUMPS

Mid-thigh Amputation: Note that bandage must be anchored around patient's waist.

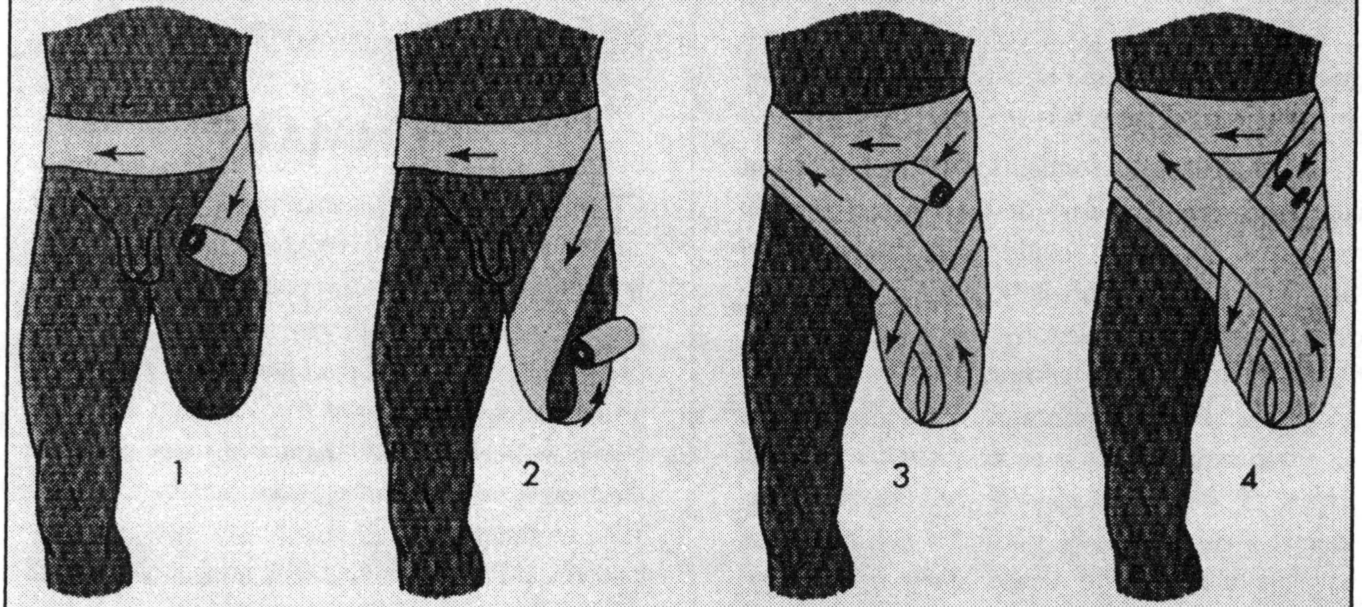

Mid-calf Amputation: Note that bandage need not be anchored around the waist.

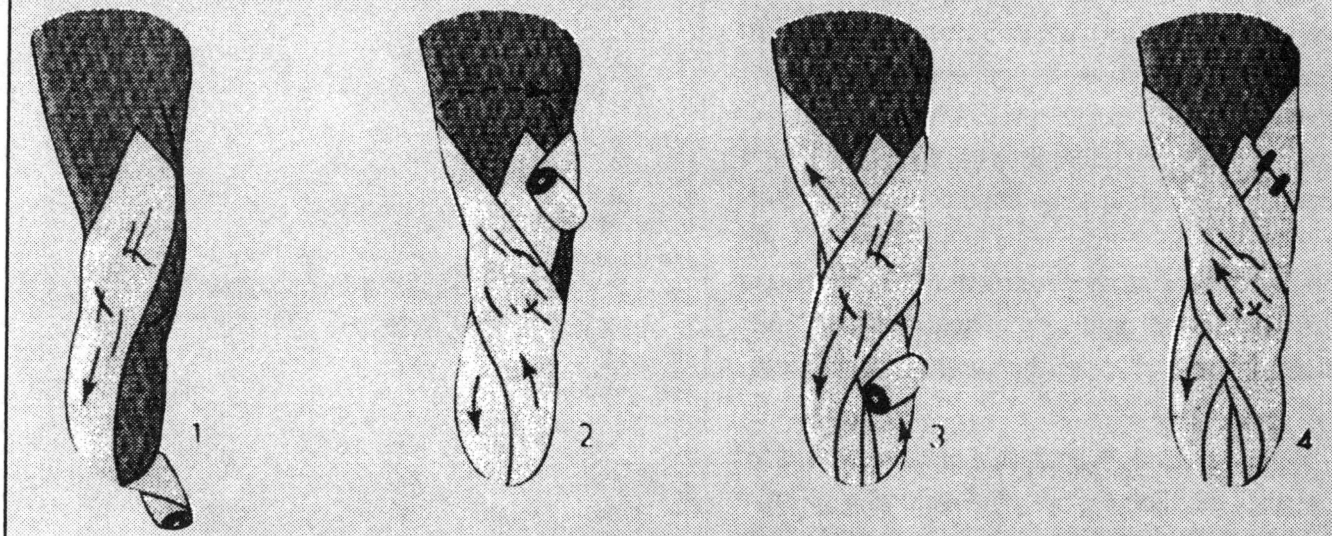

From Phipps, W., Sands, J., & Marek, J. (1999). *Medical surgical nursing: Concepts and clinical practice* (6th ed., p. 772). St. Louis, MO: Mosby. Reprinted with permission from Elsevier.

While the patient is awaiting the fitting of the prosthesis, it is important that upper body strength and flexibility be maintained or increased through range-of-motion exercises and muscle strengthening activities. Initial ambulation will require crutch walking as the patient adapts to the prosthesis. The patient will resume ambulation gradually as the limb adjusts to the presence of the prosthesis. Weight-bearing on the residual limb will also be limited initially while the wound is still new and the skin is sensitive. The length of time the patient ambulates with the prosthesis will be increased gradually as the patient's strength increases and the residual limb becomes less sensitive to pressure.

As the patient is readied for discharge, patient education about the care of the residual limb is important. The nurse should teach the patient to visually inspect the limb daily, looking for any redness or irritation caused by the prosthesis. The patient should also be instructed in the signs and symptoms of wound infection. The patient should not place the prosthesis over an irritated or infected portion of skin. If irritation or infection develops, patients should promptly notify the physician. The limb should be carefully washed daily and kept dry. Lotions should not be applied. Residual limb socks should be clean and in good repair.

A prosthetist will fit the patient with the prosthesis and instruct the patient in how to care for it. Proper care of the prosthesis will extend its life and result in a safer gait for the patient. The patient must be instructed to seek alterations of the prosthesis as necessary to maintain a good fit that does not irritate the residual limb. Adjustments to the prosthesis will probably be necessary over the next 6–12 months as the residual limb gradually changes shape. If the patient is a child, the prosthesis will require adjustment as the child grows.

Adjusting to an amputation can be difficult for many patients. There is a body-image change and it is normal for the patient to grieve the loss of a limb. The patient may feel a loss of independence and become depressed. The nurse should acknowledge the patient's feelings and refer the patient to counseling and other community resources where the patient can find support. An amputee support group may be a benefit to the patient if one exists in the community. The patient should be encouraged to be an active participant in all care, performing activities of daily living as capable. The patient should also be encouraged to assume responsibility for limb care as soon as possible, to adjust to handling the limb. With encouragement and support, most patients adapt well and live productive lives.

SUMMARY

This chapter has addressed the nursing care related to patients who have been diagnosed with a bone neoplasm. The survival outlook for those patients who have a primary malignant bone neoplasm is more hopeful than previously. Aggressive chemotherapy has altered the outcomes for many young individuals. This chapter has also addressed the nursing care of a patient who has experienced an AK amputation. The nurse can provide these patients and their families with a great deal of support as they cope with a life-threatening illness and alterations in their lifestyles.

EXAM QUESTIONS

CHAPTER 15
Questions 96-100

96. A patient who has a benign bone neoplasm, an osteoma, in his femur should be told that the tumor will likely

    a. metastasize to other organs.
    b. be well-defined in size.
    c. grow quickly and aggressively.
    d. invade the surrounding tissues.

97. A primary malignant bone neoplasm typically manifests clinically with

    a. localized pain.
    b. decreased serum calcium.
    c. paresthesia.
    d. joint deformities.

98. The treatment of choice for managing osteosarcoma is

    a. amputation of the affected extremity.
    b. radiation therapy.
    c. chemotherapy and surgical excision.
    d. bone marrow transplant.

99. The primary focus of nursing care for a patient with a malignant bone neoplasm is

    a. preventing a pathological fracture in the affected extremity.
    b. supporting the patient through the grieving process.
    c. teaching the patient how to safely use ambulatory devices.
    d. providing effective pain control.

100. Positioning a patient following an above knee amputation should involve

    a. avoiding side-lying positions.
    b. encouraging the patient to lie prone at periodic intervals.
    c. keeping the head of the bed elevated in a semi-Fowler's position.
    d. placing the residual limb on a pillow for support.

This concludes the final examination.

GLOSSARY

abduction: To move away from the midline of the body.

adduction: To move toward the midline of the body.

allograft: Bone and tissue that is provided by a donor.

autograft: Bone and tissue that is provided by the individual and transplanted to another body area.

amphiarthrotic joint: A joint that allows only limited movement.

arthrocentesis: Procedure that allows for fluid aspiration from a joint.

arthrodesis: The surgical fixation, or fusion, of a joint so that the joint is no longer movable.

arthrogram: Radiology procedure of a joint using contrast media.

arthroplasty: Joint replacement.

arthroscopy: Procedure where an endoscope is inserted into a joint for visualization of interior joint structures.

atonic: Lack of muscle tone; flaccid.

atrophy: Decrease in size; wasting away, as in atrophy of muscle mass.

avascular necrosis: A condition that develops when the femoral neck is fractured, disrupting the blood supply to the femoral head and leading to the death of the bone. A complication of femoral neck hip fractures.

ball and socket joint: A type of diarthrodial or synovial joint that allows free movement within the joint. The "ball" or rounded end of a bone fits into the "socket" or cup portion of the joint. The hip is an example of a ball and socket joint.

bone densitometry: A noninvasive diagnostic test that measures the density of the bone. Used to detect thinning of bone mass that may be indicative of osteoporosis.

Bryant's traction: Form of running skin traction used to immobilize hip joints or reduce femoral fractures in young children. The traction is attached overhead to a spreader bar on the child's legs, lifting the buttocks off of the bed.

Buck's traction: A form of running skin traction that is applied to lower extremities, most commonly to immobilize hip fractures or dislocations.

bursa: Fluid-filled sacs located throughout the body to reduce friction between body structures such as muscles or tendons and bones as movement is produced. Bursa can be found in joints such as the shoulder, elbow, hips and knees, as well as multiple other locations.

bursitis: Inflammation of the bursa, usually due to excessive use of a joint.

callus: Callus is the loose formation of newly woven bone that develops around the bone ends of a fracture during the early phases of bone healing. The presence of callus indicates that bone healing has been initiated. The callus is eventually replaced by true bone as healing continues.

cancellous bone: A structural form of bone that has a spongy, trabecular appearance. Cancellous bone is light weight and frequently lies under compact bone. Cancellous bone is also found in the epiphyses of the long bones.

carpal tunnel syndrome: Syndrome caused by the compression of the median nerve in the carpal tunnel leading to numbness and tingling in the fingers and hand. Usually caused by frequent use of wrist (repetitive motion); may also be associated with arthritis.

cartilage: Elastic, tough tissue that covers the ends of the long bones and provides a smooth articulation surface between the bone ends.

cast: A rigid form of dressing that encircles and encases an affected body part to promote immobilization of the part and maintain alignment of body structures to promote healing. Casts are made either of synthetic materials that harden quickly after application or of plaster of Paris.

cervical skin traction: A form of running skin traction that is applied to the cervical area using a soft cervical collar with weights and a pulley. Used to treat muscles spasms and nerve compression in the cervical region.

circumduction: The circular movement of an extremity. Ball and socket joints such as the hip and shoulder are capable of circumduction.

closed fracture: Fracture that does not result in a break in skin integrity; also called simple fracture.

comminuted fracture: A fractured bone that has been broken into multiple small pieces.

compact bone: Dense bone that provides a protective covering over cancellous bone in the short bones and flat bones, as well as other types of bone. Compact bone can also be found in the shafts of the long bones. Also known as cortical bone.

compartment syndrome: A syndrome in which increasing pressure is placed upon circulation, nerves, and tissues located within a given muscle compartment, leading to a decrease in blood flow through the compartment and ischemic damage to tissues and nerves. If pressure is not alleviated quickly, necrosis and permanent damage to the tissues can result in a loss of function in the affected muscle and extremity.

compound fracture: A fracture in which the skin has been broken by the fractured ends of the bone. Also known as an open fracture or a complex fracture.

continuous passive motion (CPM) device: A device that supports a joint and repetitively and passively moves the joint through range-of-motion exercises. Commonly used postoperatively for total knee replacements, a CPM device increases the range of motion in preparation for ambulation and decreases formation of edema following surgery.

contracture: Abnormal shortening of a muscle resulting in deformity of the affected joint. Can result in a permanent disability. Contractures can develop as a result of a disease process (such as rheumatoid arthritis) or can be the result of improper positioning and lack of joint exercise and movement. Range-of-motion exercises and proper positioning of a joint can prevent many contractures from forming.

cortical bone: Dense bone that provides a protective covering over cancellous bone in the short bones and flat bones, as well as other types of bone. Cortical bone can also be found in the shafts of the long bones. Also known as compact bone.

crepitus: A grating sound or sensation that occurs in a joint that has lost the smooth articulation of cartilage or bone ends of a fracture rubbing together.

delayed union: Delayed healing of bone fracture ends.

diaphysis: The shaft of a long bone

diarthrodial joint: A joint that is freely movable.

dislocation: The displacement of a bone end from its correct position in a joint. Results in pain, deformity of the joint, and loss of function.

edema: The accumulation of excess fluid in tissue, resulting in swelling.

effusion: A collection of fluid in a body part. Joint effusion may develop as a result of injury, inflammation, or infection.

epiphyseal growth plate: The portion of the long bone, located between the epiphyses and the diaphysis, that allows for the longitudinal growth of children. As individuals age to adulthood, the epiphyseal growth plate calcifies, signaling the end of the growth of the extremity.

epiphyses: The ends of long bones.

extension: The movement of a joint that ends with the joint forming a straight line.

external fixation: The process by which a bone fracture is immobilized and fixated externally through the use of metal pins, screws, etc. inserted into the bone. Usually used with fractures that are accompanied by soft tissue injuries that require treatment. May also be used to stabilize pelvic fractures.

eversion: The process of turning outward; as in the eversion of the foot.

fascia: Fibrous tissue that lies over muscles and organs.

fasciotomy: An incision into skeletal muscle fascia to relieve pressure on vascular and nerve structures.

flaccid: Term frequently applied to muscles; lacking in tone.

flexion: The movement of a joint that results in the joint being bent.

fracture: A break in a bone resulting in the disruption of the bones' continuity.

gliding joint: A type of diarthrodial or synovial joint in which the bone ends are relatively flat and glide against each other to produce movement. Movement in gliding joints is minimal. Small bones in the wrist form one example of a gliding joint.

gout: A type of arthritis that is caused by an excess of uric acid in the blood. Uric acid crystals are deposited in the joints causing an inflammation of the joint.

haversian system: The structural unit of compact bone.

hemiarthrosis: Blood in the joint cavity

hinge joint: Hinge joints are diarthrodial or synovial joints in which joint movement is limited to flexion and extension (forward and backward, as in a hinge). The elbow and knee are examples of a hinge joint.

hypertrophy: Enlargement of tissues or organs due to enlarged cells; frequently used in reference to muscles.

hyperuricemia: Elevated uric acid levels in the blood.

inversion: The process of turning inward; as in the inversion of the foot.

involucrum: Present in osteomyelitis, involucrum is a layer of new bone that grows around the sequestrum, thus surrounding the infected bone tissue.

isometric exercises: Active exercises in which muscles maintain length, muscle tension is increased, and no joint movement is produced.

isotonic exercises: Active exercise in which muscles maintain equal tension, muscle shortens, and joint movement is produced.

joint: The meeting of two or more bones.

joint capsule: Also referred to as an articular capsule. The joint capsule encloses synovial joints.

kyphosis: Increase convex spinal curvature in the thoracic area; commonly caused by osteoporosis.

ligament: Band of fibrous tissue that connects bones, providing support to joints.

logroll: Method of turning patient while maintaining spinal alignment.

lordosis: Increased concave spinal curvature in the lumbar area.

malunion: A union of the bone ends that is not properly aligned.

manipulation: Forceful movement of joint or fracture to correct (or reduce) a misalignment of structures.

meniscus: Crescent-shaped fibrous cartilage that is located in the knee joint.

metaphysis: The wider part of a long bone, located between the epiphysis and diaphysis.

myelogram: A radiology procedure of the spinal cord involving the injection of contrast medium into the subarachnoid space.

neurovascular status: Pertains to the status of the nerves and blood vessels of affected body parts, typically extremities following a musculoskeletal injury or surgery. Nursing assessment of the neurovascular status of an affected body part includes assessment of pulses, temperature, sensation, movement, and color.

nonunion: Bony fragments do not reunite following a fracture; healing of the fracture does not occur.

open reduction with internal fixation (ORIF): Surgical intervention to reduce a fracture and stabilize the reduction with the insertion of metal pins, screws and plates, or nails.

orthosis: Term for orthopedic appliances such as braces or splints. Orthoses (plural).

ossification: The formation of bone.

osteoarthritis: Also known as degenerative joint disease; a form of arthritis that is non-systemic and non-inflammatory, resulting in the degeneration of the articular cartilage.

osteoblast: A cell which produces bone.

osteoclast: A cell which participates in the resorption of bone.

osteocyte: A mature osteoblast cell within the bone matrix.

osteon: The basic structural unit of compact bone.

osteogenesis: The process of bone formation.

osteomyelitis: Infection of a bone; may be acute or chronic.

osteoporosis: A bone disorder caused by the decrease of bone mass or density; most common in postmenopausal women.

Paget's Disease: Another term for osteitis deformans, a chronic skeletal disease that results in thickening of the long bones and deformity of the flat bones.

pannus: Inflammatory synovial tissue that develops in rheumatoid arthritis.

paralysis: Loss of motor function.

paresthesia: Abnormal sensation in a body part, such as a tingling or burning feeling.

pathologic fracture: Fracture that occurs as a result of another pathological process, such as a neoplasm.

pelvic traction: A form of running skin traction periodically applied to the lower back region to treat muscle spasms or nerve impairment in the lower back.

periosteum: A connective tissue that covers the bones.

photophobia: Sensitivity of the eyes to light.

pivot joint: A synovial joint in which one bone moves around in a circular fashion allowing for rotation. The joint that allows for movement between the first and second cervical vertebrae is an example of a pivot joint.

pronation: The process of turning the palm of the hand downward by medially rotating the forearm.

reduction: The correction of a fracture in which realignment of the bone ends is achieved.

remodeling: Refers to the process of bone resorption and formation so that bone is reshaped into a functional form. This process is a dynamic one that in normal bone remains in balance.

rheumatoid arthritis: A chronic systemic, inflammatory disease that attacks connective tissue in the body, most commonly affecting the joints.

residual limb: Following an amputation of an extremity, the viable remainder of the extremity over which a prosthetic limb may be placed.

rotation: The process of turning on an axis.

Rotator cuff: Refers to the shoulder muscles and associated tendons: supraspinatus, infraspinatus, subscapularis, and teres minor.

Russell's traction: A form of balanced suspension skin traction that is used to treat distal femoral fractures in the lower extremity. Russell's traction employs the use of a popliteal knee sling to provide slight flexion to the knee, which predisposes the patient to the development of deep vein thrombosis.

saddle joint: A synovial joint that allows for easy movement in a multitude of directions. The base of the thumb is an example of a saddle joint.

sciatica: Pain that radiates down the sciatica nerve causing pain in the back of the thigh down to the foot.

scoliosis: Lateral curvature of the spine; occurs more commonly in girls.

sequestrum: An area of dead bone. Sequestrum develops in osteomyelitis as a result of infection.

simple fracture: Another term for closed fracture.

skeletal muscle: Striated muscle attached to bones that produce movement.

skeletal traction: Traction that is applied to realign a fractured bone by applying weights to a pin or wire that has been surgically inserted into the bone. The weight of the traction is applied directly to the bone. Fractured femur is an example of a fracture that is frequently treated by the application of skeletal traction.

skin traction: Traction that is indirectly applied to a dislocated joint or fractured bone through the application of a bandage (such as an ace wrap) to the affected extremity that holds the traction in place. Skin traction is usually a temporary form of treatment, frequently used to immobilize a fracture until surgery can be performed.

spastic: Tightening of muscles due to increased tension.

sprain: Ligament injury at a joint.

strain: A pull or tear in a skeletal muscle.

supination: The process of turning the palm upward by laterally rotating the forearm.

synarthrotic joint: Also known as a fibrous or immovable joint, in which the bone ends are connected by fibrous tissue allowing minimal motion.

synovial fluid: Fluid that is secreted by the synovium into the joint capsule; serves as a lubricant and shock absorber.

synovial joint: Joint that allows free movement between bone ends which are encased in a joint capsule. Also referred to as a diarthrodial joint.

subluxation: A partial dislocation of a joint.

tendon: Fibrous tissue that connects the end of a muscle to a bone; allows the muscle to produce movement.

tendonitis: Inflammation of a tendon.

tone: The tension present within a muscle.

tophi: An accumulation of uric acid crystal deposits in a joint. Tophi develop in gout.

traction: The application of a pulling force that is used to achieve and maintain proper alignment of a dislocated joint or fractured bone ends so that healing may occur. May also be used to overcome muscle spasms (as in lower back pain) or to prevent or decrease the development of contractures.

Volkmann's contracture: Contracture of the fingers and wrist as the result of restricted blood flow caused by compartment syndrome.

BIBLIOGRAPHY

Ahearn-Spera, M. (2000). Assessment of neurological function. In S. Smeltzer & B. Bare (Eds.), *Brunner & Suddarth's textbook of medical-surgical nursing* (pp. 1608–1632). Philadelphia: Lippincott Williams & Wilkins.

Altizer, L. (2002). Neurovascular assessment. *Orthopaedic Nursing, 21*(4), 48–50.

Andres, B., Mears, S., & Wenz, J. (2001). Surgical treatment options for cartilage defects within the knee. *Orthopaedic Nursing, 20*(3), 27–31.

Ayello, E. & Perry, A. (2001). Skin integrity and wound care. In P. Potter & A. Perry (Eds.), *Fundamentals of nursing* (5th ed., pp. 1545–1629). St.Louis: Mosby.

Bender, C., Yasko, J., & Strohl, R. (2000). Cancer. In S. M. Lewis, M. M. Heitkemper, & S. R. Dirksen (Eds.), *Medical-surgical nursing: Assessment and management of clinical problems* (5th ed., pp. 269-322). St. Louis: Mosby.

Black, J., Hawks, J., & Keene, A. (2001). *Medical-surgical nursing: Clinical management of positive outcomes* (6th ed.). Philadelphia, PA: WB Saunders Co.

Bush, M. (2000). Arthritis and other rheumatic disorders. In S. M. Lewis, M. M. Heitkemper, & S. R. Dirksen (Eds.), *Medical-surgical nursing: Assessment and management of clinical problems* (5th ed., pp. 1819–1861). St. Louis: Mosby.

Byrne, T. (1999). The setup and care of a patient in Buck's traction. *Orthopaedic Nursing, 18*(2), 79–83.

Casteel, K. (2003). Musculoskeletal assessment. In J. Weber & J. Kelley (Eds.). *Health assessment in nursing* (2nd ed., pp. 497–539). Philadelphia: Lippincott Williams & Wilkins.

Childs, S. G. (2002). Pathogenesis of anterior cruciate ligament injury. *Orthopaedic Nursing, 21*(4), 35–40.

Dingley, C. (1999). Disorders of the musculoskeletal system. In C. Reeves, G. Roux, & R. Lockhart (Eds.), *Medical-surgical nursing* (pp. 233–276). St. Louis: McGraw-Hill.

Ditmyer, M., Topp, R., & Pifer, M. (2002). Prehabilitation in preparation for orthopaedic surgery. *Orthopaedic Nursing, 21*(5), 43–53.

Doheny, M. & Sedlak, C. (2001). Assessment of the musculoskeletal system. In J. Black, J. Hawks, & A. Keene (Eds.), *Medical surgical nursing: Clinical management for positive outcomes* (pp. 537–549). Philadelphia: Saunders.

Eggenberger, S. (1998). Knowledge base for patients with musculoskeletal dysfunction. In F. Monahan & M. Neighbors (Eds.), *Medical-surgical nursing: Foundations for clinical practice* (2nd ed., pp. 837–886). Philadelphia: W. B. Saunders.

Feldt, K. & Finch, M. (2002). Older adults with hip fractures: Treatment of pain following hospitalization. *Journal of Gerontological Nursing, 28*(8), 27–35.

Feldt, K. & Gunderson, J. (2002). Treatment of pain for older hip fracture patients across settings. *Orthopaedic Nursing, 21*(5), 63–71.

Fried, K. M. & Fried, G. (2001). Immobility. In J. Derstine & S. Hargrove (Eds.), *Comprehensive rehabilitation nursing.* Philadelphia: W.B. Saunders Co., pp. 163–169.

Geier, K. A.(2001). Osteoporosis in men. *Orthopaedic Nursing, 20*(6), 49–56.

Gordon, D.B. (1998). Assessment and management of pain. In A. Maher, S. Salmond, & T. Pellino (Eds.), *Orthopedic Nursing* (pp. 115–144). Philadelphia: W.B. Saunders.

Hargrove, S. D. & Derstine, J.B. (2001). Definition and philosophy of rehabilitation nursing: History and scope including chronicity and disability. In J. Derstine & S. Hargrove (Eds.), *Comprehensive rehabilitation nursing* (pp. 3–10). Philadelphia: W.B. Saunders.

Jagmin, M. G. (1998). Assessment and management of immobility. In A. Maher, S. Salmond, & T. Pellino (Eds.), *Orthopedic Nursing,* (pp. 92–114). Philadelphia: W.B. Saunders.

Kotch, M. J. (2001). Nursing management of the patient with an orthopedic disorder. In J. Derstine & S. Hargrove (Eds.), *Comprehensive rehabilitation nursing,* (pp. 424–463). Philadelphia: W.B. Saunders.

Kunkler, C. E. (1999). Neurovascular assessment. *Orthopaedic Nursing, 18*(3), 63–71.

Lamb, K. & Cummings, M. (2000). Musculoskeletal function. In A. Lueckenotte (Ed.), *Gerontologic Nursing* (2nd ed., pp. 721–756). St. Louis: Mosby.

LeMone, P. & Burke, K. (2004) *Medical surgical nursing: Critical thinking in client care* (3rd ed.) Englewood Cliffs, NJ: Prentice-Hall.

Lewis, S., Heitkemper, M., & Dirksen, S. (2000). *Medical-surgical nursing: Assessment and management of clinical problems* (5th ed.). St. Louis, MO: Mosby.

Liddel, D. B. (2000a). Assessment of musculoskeletal function. In S. Smeltzer & B. Bare (Eds.), *Brunner & Suddarth's textbook of medical-surgical nursing* (pp. 1764–1777). Philadelphia: Lippincott Williams & Wilkins.

Liddel, D. B. (2000b). Management of patients with musculoskeletal trauma. In S. Smeltzer & B. Bare (Eds). *Brunner & Suddarth's textbook of medical-surgical nursing* (9th ed., pp. 1831–1865). Philadelphia: Lippincott Williams & Wilkins.

Liddel, D. B. (2000c). Musculoskeletal care modalities. In S. Smeltzer & B. Bare (Eds.), *Brunner & Suddarth's textbook of medical-surgical nursing* (9th ed., pp. 1779–1805). Philadelphia: Lippincott Williams & Wilkins.

Lundon, K. (2000). Metabolic bone disease. In K. Lundon (Ed.), *Orthopedic rehabilitation science: Principles for clinical management of bone* (pp. 155–185). Boston: Butterworth-Heinemann.

MacDonald, V. & Hilton, B. A. (2001). Postoperative pain management in frail older adults. *Orthopaedic Nursing, 20*(3), 63–76.

Marek, J. F. (1999a). Assessment of the musculoskeletal system. In W. J. Phipps, J. K. Sands, & J. F. Marek (Eds.), *Medical-surgical nursing: Concepts & clinical practice* (6th ed., pp. 1881–1913). St. Louis: Mosby.

Marek, J. F. (1999b). Management of persons with trauma to the musculoskeletal system. In W. J. Phipps, J. K. Sands, & J. F. Marek (Eds.), *Medical-surgical nursing: Concepts & clinical practice* (6th ed., pp. 1915–1955). St. Louis: Mosby.

McCance, K. L. & Mourad, L. A. (2000). Alterations of musculoskeletal function. In S. E. Huether & K. L. McCance (Eds.), *Understanding pathophysiology* (2nd ed., pp. 1031–1073). St. Louis: Mosby.

Milisen, K., Foreman, M., Wouters, B., Driesen, R., Godderis, J., Abraham, I.L. et al. (2002). Documentation of delirium in elderly patients with hip fracture. *Journal of Gerontological Nursing, 28*(11), 23–9.

Mourad, L. A. (2000). Structure and function of the musculoskeletal system. In S. E. Huether & K. L. McCance (Eds.), *Understanding pathophysiology* (2nd ed., pp. 1007–1030). St. Louis: Mosby.

National Institute of Arthritis and Musculoskeletal and Skin Diseases (NIAMS) (1999). Handout on Health: Rheumatoid Arthritis. Retrieved April 2, 2004 from http://www.niams.nih.gov/hi/topics/arthritis/rahandout.htm#ra_5

Phipps, W., Sands, J., & Marek, J. (1999). *Medical surgical nursing: Concepts and clinical practice* (6th ed.). St. Louis, MO: Mosby.

Pigg, J. S. (2000). Management of patients with rheumatic disorders. In S. Smeltzer & B. Bare (Eds.), *Brunner & Suddarth's textbook of medical-surgical nursing* (9th ed., pp. 1405–1433). Philadelphia: Lippincott Williams & Wilkins.

Potter, P. & Perry, A. (2000). Fundamentals of Nursing (5th ed.). St. Louis: Mosby.

Rice, K. L. & Walsh, E. (2001). Minimizing venous thromboembolic complications in the orthopaedic patient. *Orthopaedic Nursing, 20*(6), 21–27.

Roberts, D. (2001). Management of clients with musculoskeletal trauma or overuse. In J. Black, J. Hawks, & A. Keene (Eds.), *Medical surgical nursing: Clinical management for positive outcomes* (pp. 587–625). Philadelphia: Saunders.

Roberts, D. & Lappe, J. (2001). Management of clients with musculoskeletal disorders. In J. Black, J. Hawks, & A. Keene (Eds.), *Medical surgical nursing: Clinical management for positive outcomes* (pp. 551–585). Philadelphia: Saunders.

Ruda, S. C. (2000a). Nursing assessment: Musculoskeletal system. In S. M. Lewis, M. M. Heitkemper, & S. R. Dirksen (Eds.), *Medical-surgical nursing: Assessment and management of clinical problems* (5th ed., pp. 1745–1761). St. Louis: Mosby.

Ruda, S. C. (2000b). Nursing management: Musculoskeletal problems. In S. M. Lewis, M. M. Heitkemper, & S. R. Dirksen (Eds.), *Medical-surgical nursing: Assessment and management of clinical problems* (5th ed., pp. 1762–1818). St. Louis: Mosby.

Schoen, D. C. (2000). *Adult orthopaedic nursing.* Philadelphia: Lippincott, Williams & Wilkins.

Stewart, K. B. (2000). Open fracture. *Nursing, 30*(11), 33.

Spotlight on orthopedic nursing. (2002). *Nursing 2002, 32*(12), 20.

Trauma.Org, The Trauma Image Bank, (n.d.). Retrieved April 14, 2004 from http://www.trauma.org/imagebank/imagebank.html

Turkoski, B. (2002). Treating osteoporosis without hormones. *Orthopaedic Nursing, 21*(5), 80–85.

Warner, C. (2001). The use of the orthopaedic perioperative autotransfusion (orthPAT-trademark) system in total joint replacement surgery. *Orthopaedic Nursing, 20*(6), 29–32.

INDEX

PRETEST KEY

Orthopedic Nursing:
Caring for Patients with Musculoskeletal Disorders

1.	b	Chapter 2
2.	c	Chapter 2
3.	c	Chapter 3
4.	b	Chapter 3
5.	d	Chapter 7
6.	d	Chapter7
7.	a	Chapter 7
8.	c	Chapter 8
9.	a	Chapter8
10.	d	Chapter 10
11.	b	Chapter 13
12.	c	Chapter 4
13.	a	Chapter 6
14.	b	Chapter 7
15.	c	Chapter 7
16.	a	Chapter 8
17.	b	Chapter 9
18.	b	Chapter 9
19.	c	Chapter 12
20.	d	Chapter 14
21.	b	Chapter 1
22.	b	Chapter 5
23.	a	Chapter 11
24.	c	Chapter 15

Western Schools® offers over 60 topics to suit all your interests – and requirements!

Clinical Conditions/Nursing Practice

A Nurse's Guide to Weight Control
for Healthy Living.............................25 hrs
Auscultation Skills: Breath and Heart Sounds ......12 hrs
Basic Nursing of Head, Chest, Abdominal,
Spine and Orthopedic Trauma ....16 hrs
Care at the End of Life...............................3 hrs
Chest Tube Management ....2 hrs
Diabetes Nursing Care...............................30 hrs
Healing Nutrition ....24 hrs
Hepatitis C: The Silent Killer ....2 hrs
HIV/AIDS.............................1, 2, 4 or 30 hrs
Holistic & Complementary Therapies: Introduction..1 hr
Influenza: A Vaccine-Preventable Disease ....1 hr
Managing Obesity and Eating Disorders ....30 hrs
Orthopedic Nursing: Caring for Patients with
Musculoskeletal Disorders ....30 hrs
Pain Management: Principles and Practice............30 hrs
Popular Diets and Diet Drugs ....2 hrs
Practical Weight Control: Assessment & Planning..7 hrs
Practical Weight Control: Lifestyle Interventions..10 hrs
Pressure Ulcers: Guidelines for Prevention
and Nursing Management...............................30 hrs
The Neurological Exam...............................1 hr
Wound Management and Healing.......................30 hrs

Cosmetic Treatments/Surgery

Belt Lipectomy: Lower Body Contouring ....1 hr
Botox Treatments and Dermal Fillers.................1 hr
Cosmetic Breast Surgery ....1 hr
Weight Loss Surgery ....1 hr

Critical Care/ER/OR

Ambulatory Surgical Care ....20 hrs
Case Studies in Critical Care Nursing:
A Guide for Application and Review ....36 hrs
Principles of Basic Trauma Nursing ....30 hrs

Geriatrics

Alzheimer's: Things a Nurse Needs to Know........12 hrs
Elder Abuse ....4 hrs
Home Health Nursing ....30 hrs
Major Issues in Gerontological Nursing ....10 hrs
Nursing Care of the Older Adult ....30 hrs

Infectious Diseases/Bioterrorism

Biological Weapons ....5 hrs
Bioterrorism & the Nurse's Response to WMD ......5 hrs
Influenza: A Vaccine-Preventable Disease ....1 hr
SARS: An Emerging Public Health Threat ....1 hr
Smallpox..2 hrs
The New Threat of Drug Resistant Microbes ....5 hrs
West Nile Virus ....1 hr

Maternal-Child/Pediatrics/Women's Health

Attention Deficit Hyperactivity Disorders
Throughout the Lifespan...............................30 hrs
Challenges in Women's Health: PMS;
Reproductive Choices; Menopause;
Gynecological Disorders ....2-5 hrs
End-of-Life Care for Children and
Their Families ....2 hrs
IPV (Intimate Partner Violence):
A Domestic Violence Concern ....1 or 3 hrs
Manual of School Health...............................30 hrs
Maternal-Newborn Nursing..............................30 hrs
Pediatric Nursing: Routine to Emergent Care........30 hrs
Pediatric Pharmacology...............................10 hrs
Pediatric Physical Assessment........................10 hrs
Women's Health: Contemporary
Advances and Trends ....30 hrs

Oncology

Cancer in Women......................................30 hrs
Cancer Nursing: A Solid Foundation for Practice ..30 hrs
Chemotherapy Essentials: Principles & Practice ..15 hrs

Professional Issues/Management/Law

Medical Error Prevention: Patient Safety ....2 hrs
Nursing Ethics and the Law...........................30 hrs
Nursing and Malpractice Risks:
Understanding the Law................................30 hrs
Ohio Law: Standards of Safe Nursing Practice ....1 hr
Supervisory Skills for Nurses ....30 hrs
Surviving and Thriving in Nursing ....30 hrs
Understanding Managed Care...........................30 hrs

Psychiatric/Mental Health

Basic Psychopharmacology.............................5 hrs
Child Abuse ....30 hrs
IPV (Intimate Partner Violence):
A Domestic Violence Concern ....1 or 3 hrs
Psychiatric Principles & Applications for
General Patient Care ....30 hrs
Psychiatric Nursing Update: Current Trends
in Diagnosing and Treatment ....30 hrs
Substance Abuse ....30 hrs

**For our free catalog, visit our website
www.westernschools.com
or call today!**

1-800-438-8888

Visit us online at www.westernschools.com for these great courses – plus all the latest CE topics!
Online testing also available. REV. 4/04 v2